WELLNESS:
JUST A STATE OF MIND?

By
Eldon Taylor, Ph.D.

Foreword by
Rayford Fountain, Esq.

I dedicate this book to Roy,
in memory of my colleague, friend and business partner
who left this earth plane on June 4, 1991.

Table of Contents

Foreword iii
About the Author vii
Acknowledgments and Introduction ix
Prologue xi
1. The Adventure Begins 1
2. The Basis for Our Beliefs 3
3. My Story 7
4. A Two-Way Communication? 13
5. Some Interesting Phenomena 17
6. Personality 19
7. Stress 23
8. Conditioning 29
9. What We Expect Is What We Get 33
10. A Trip Down Memory Lane 41
11. The Power of Belief 45
12. The Pragmatist Within 47
13. The Scientist Emerges 53
14. Owning Your Own Controls 57
15. Making It All Work 69
16. The Seven Fundamentals 73
Epilogue 87
Recommended Readings 99
Appendix A 102

Foreword

One of the most frustrating endeavors for a person not trained in science is to try to wade through a book written by a scientist who has no perspective of the lay-person's point of view. Fortunately, in this book which you are about to read, Dr. Eldon Taylor has done a wonderful job of discussing complex scientific theories that have to do with the mechanical structure of the mind and body, as well as the psychological and behavioral aspects of the human personality in a "down-to-earth" and "common-sense" style which makes it understandable to the average person.

Sadly, the fact is that many lay people (and unfortunately many doctors) still approach the mind-body paradigm according to Newtonian mechanical physics. To many people "man" means simply the "mechanical man." The truth is: we live in a new age where the leading scientists in many different disciplines are now understanding the human body and personality in terms of the "new physics." There is a plethora of evidence in both the study of physics and metaphysics that the human being is not just a mechanical creature, but is a creature that can be truly understood only if one takes into account the complete "holistic" aspect of his or her being.

Dr. Eldon Taylor is a person who is uniquely qualified to approach the task he set out for himself in writing this book. Not only is Dr. Taylor a renowned scientist in his field of expertise, but he possesses a deep personal sense of the "spiritual" and metaphysical aspects of the human condition. There are a great deal of phenomena (particularly concerning wellness, sickness and healing) that cannot be explained by strict scientific analysis. As more is being learned about the mind-body connection and the value of "holistic" approaches to health and wellness, we are finding that what was once relegated to New Age metaphysics is now becoming the accepted physics.

This latest book by Dr. Taylor will lead you on an exciting and interesting journey explaining the connection between your mind, thinking and attitudes and how they absolutely affect your state of well-being and health. We all want to stay healthy and well and the super-exciting discovery is that your wellness is pretty much up to you--it really is all a state of your mind.

I want to take this opportunity to thank my good friend, Dr. Eldon Taylor, for bringing the message of this book to all of us in a clear and simple fashion which is easily digestible by the layman and will improve all of our lives. The only real purpose in life is to be happy--and it is tough to be happy if you are not well.

Rayford Fountain, Esq.
Pasadena, California

Mr. Fountain is a practicing trial attorney. He also is the founder of the Big Bear Center for Creative Living in Big Bear City, California. This organization is dedicated to helping people achieve greater awareness, spiritual growth and harmony in their lives.

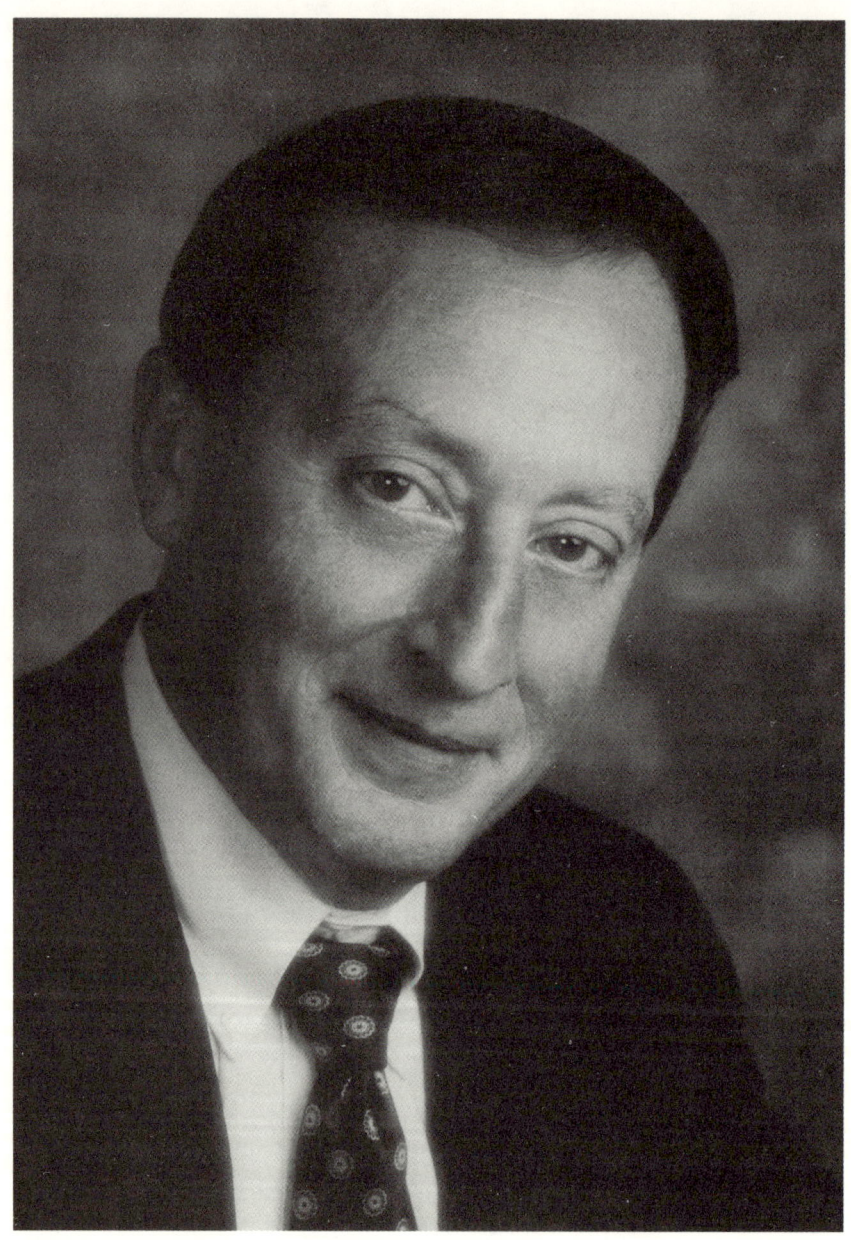

About the Author

Eldon Taylor is president of Progressive Awareness Research, an organization dedicated to researching alternative techniques to facilitate self empowerment. For many years he was an investigator, who specialized in psycho-physical feedback such as lie detection testing.

Today, Eldon describes himself as a sort of cowboy philosopher whose favorite endeavors include science, philosophy, poetry and horse breeding. He believes that life is a school, and that the human condition is inherently endowed with the absolute power and ability to enjoy and utilize much vaster potential than is currently even dreamed of by many. As a pragmatist his work emphasizes the use of science and philosophy as opposed to the theory. The statement, "If it doesn't work, all the theories in the world have little or no value!" sums up his basic belief.

Considered to be one of the world's leading authorities on subliminal information processing, Eldon has lectured in the United Kingdom, Germany, Hong Kong and the United States. His work with subliminal communication has been translated into five languages. It was featured by *Omni* in their anniversary audio experience issue and has been referred to in numerous newspapers and magazines.

Eldon has written eight books and more than two hundred audio cassette programs. His work with behavioral medicine led to the development of special audio programs for cancer, AIDS, and other diseases. Universities in the United States and Germany have proven the patented "Taylor method," or **WHOLE BRAIN**[R] technology, to be effective.

Eldon has also been distinguished in many leading *Who's Who* publications, including the prestigious *Who's Who of Intellectuals* and the *Who's Who Among Human Service Professionals*.

Eldon says he loves his work, and we hope you will, too.

Acknowledgments and Introduction

In very many ways I feel that this work is a primer of the "see Spot run" type when it comes to unraveling the mind-body connection in wellness and longevity. In other ways I am deeply gratified by the tremendous encouragement and positive feedback that led to producing this little book.

Many, many people suggested that I tell the story of wellness in simple terms that could be understood by anyone. One of my publishers, Leslie, insisted that only academicians benefitted from scientifically written papers and further, she asserted, most of the popular books in the area of the mind-body wellness connection failed to give a "how to" simple enough to put into practice. For Leslie, telling the story as a story while connecting the dots, so to speak, from the scientific literature to form a picture that all could understand and use just made sense. That is precisely the form of a **WELLNESS: JUST A STATE OF MIND?** I am indebted to Leslie both for her encouragement and for her insistence that the material be easily understood.

I am also in the debt of my editors, Ravinder Taylor and Suzanne Brady, who spent many hours assisting me in creating a form that is easily understood and also includes enough factual scientific findings to satisfy my inclination to support, support, and support each assertion.

When I became frustrated with the material, mainly because so much of what I had written was deleted, my wonderful wife Ravinder reminded me that it is what a book **does** for the reader that is important, not how many words it contains. Her encouragement to write in such a manner as to produce a process in the reader became the mandate of the material that follows. Although initially I resisted the idea of cartoons in one of my books, also one of Ravinder's ideas, when I look at the completed project I feel that the book accomplishes its objectives. For those who have read it, Ravinder's conceptualizations in cartoon form, brought to life by Richelle Bryant, who also deserves my many thanks, have stuck in their minds and often served as a catalyst to recall thoughts or ideas provoked in them while reading. These readers tell me that the book **works**! I sincerely hope that this book also works in providing added quality to your life in health, wellness in all matters, and longevity.

A special thank you is owed to my treasured friend, Rayford Fountain, for his invaluable advice and support. Additionally, I must thank two special people whose confidence, trust, and support has meant much to me in a number of endeavors, including this book--thank you Lois Bey and Pat Brown.

Last, but not least, to the many pioneering researchers who dared to tread on the sometimes sacred ground of orthodoxy, we are all indebted. Their work continues to unravel the mystery of being human in dimensions that challenge the very fiber of much of what has been called "axiomatic" by science for centuries. Without these pioneers, this book would have no context.

Eldon Taylor, Ph.D.

Prologue

by the Editor

Isn't it interesting how often science fiction becomes scientific fact? We used to think that man would never walk on the moon or sail beneath the surface of the seas. Science even used to argue that the earth was flat and that the sun and the galaxies rotated around it. Nowadays, most of us laugh at such ideas.

Knowing how frequently "science" has been proven wrong, why do so many of us still find it hard to accept the mind-body wellness connection? The idea that our minds have an amazing power over our health appears to defy much of what science has taught us. How then would you react if I told you, as a "scientific fact," that certain personalities are able to change their eye color in the time it takes to snap your fingers? Pretty amazing, don't you think?

You know, there was a time when I too would have believed that such "science fiction" could never become "scientific fact." After all, I was a trained microbiologist. However, Eldon, a former criminologist, trained in psychology, decided to use these tools and investigate every clue that might lead to a definite answer. What follows is the journey he undertook before he came to the conclusion that we absolutely **do** have control over our health, wellness, and longevity. Just how much control--I'll leave that up to you to decide.

Enjoy,

Ravinder Sadana-Taylor

There's a story I can tell . . .
about a time to feel swell.
It's as simple as this:
I expect to be well!

Chapter One

The Adventure Begins

For centuries stories have proliferated about the incredible powers of the mind, feats of mind over body that even to a child seem impossible or absurd. How, for example, can a human chew glass or hot coals and not be injured? How can a person lie on a bed of needles and not have a single needle pierce the skin? What trick is involved in fire-walking? What powers exist in the spiritual healer's touch? How do the masters of the East control breathing, heartbeat, and skin temperature? Like all the magical stories of mind and body, there are many in the area of wellness that have defied scientific inquiry, including many miraculous healings, such as those reported as the result of following the advice in the book of Matthew:

> **If you had FAITH, even as small as a tiny mustard seed . . . nothing would be impossible.**

What is the magical relationship between mind and body? Is it available to the scrutiny of science? Does it really exist, and if so, can we all learn to use it for our benefit? Can each of us enhance our health, our wellness, even perhaps our

1

longevity by using some process that the mind can control? And how much influence is really possible? Everyone knows that managing stress, a mental process, can enhance health; but can the mind change something as physical as the twisted body of one suffering from a severe bone or muscle disease?

It was questions such as these that sparked my life-long quest for insight in matters of the mind-body connection and wellness.

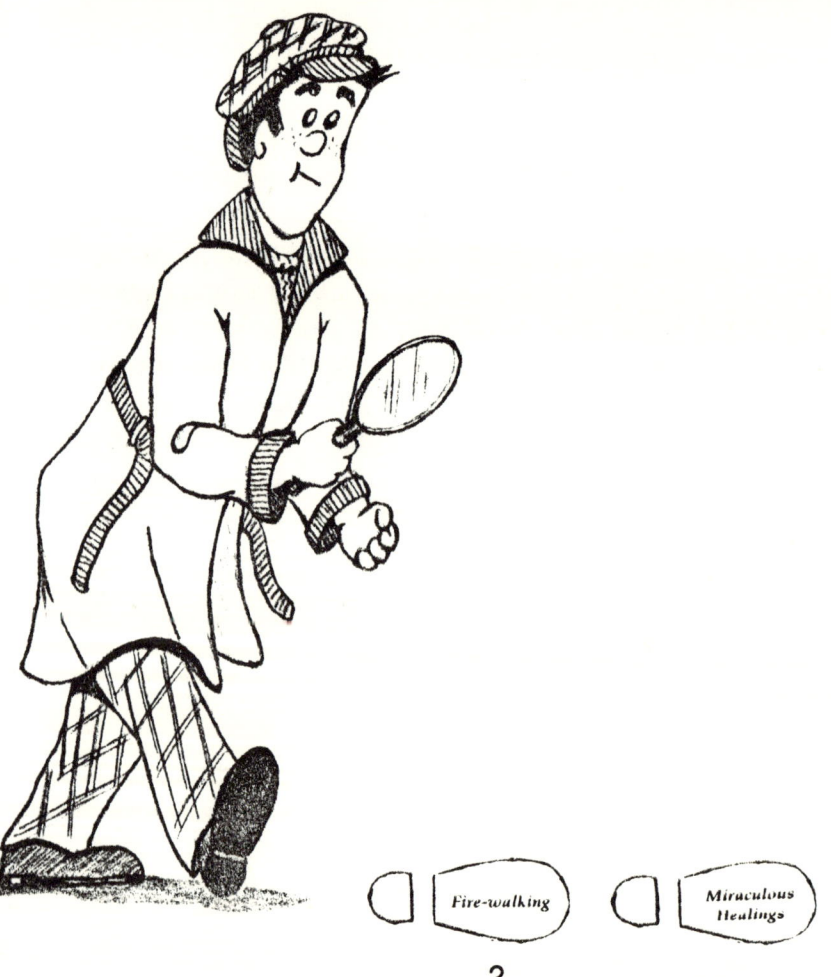

Fire-walking   Miraculous Healings

Chapter Two

The Basis for Our Beliefs

I started my investigation by examining the basis for our current beliefs in health care. It seems that as science developed, so did the idea of a mechanical man. The mind and body were considered to be separate; they functioned independently and should therefore be treated separately. This is rather like comparing the body to a machine, which depends upon the springs, gears, and what-not for both function and identity.

The body is made up of lots of cells that collectively form organs, information systems, and so on. These cells are often assumed to work like computer microchips, each with its own duties and tasks. The cell is ahead of the microchip in that it is a self-replicating system that processes the environment and uses this information to organize behavior. A cell is therefore capable of reproducing itself but, according to most, it is not conscious in the sense that it does not have an independent will. As we'll see later, this is an assumption based on purely arbitrary definitions of consciousness. After all, if the cells had consciousness, who would be doing the thinking in each of us anyway? Still, it is this idea--of the

3

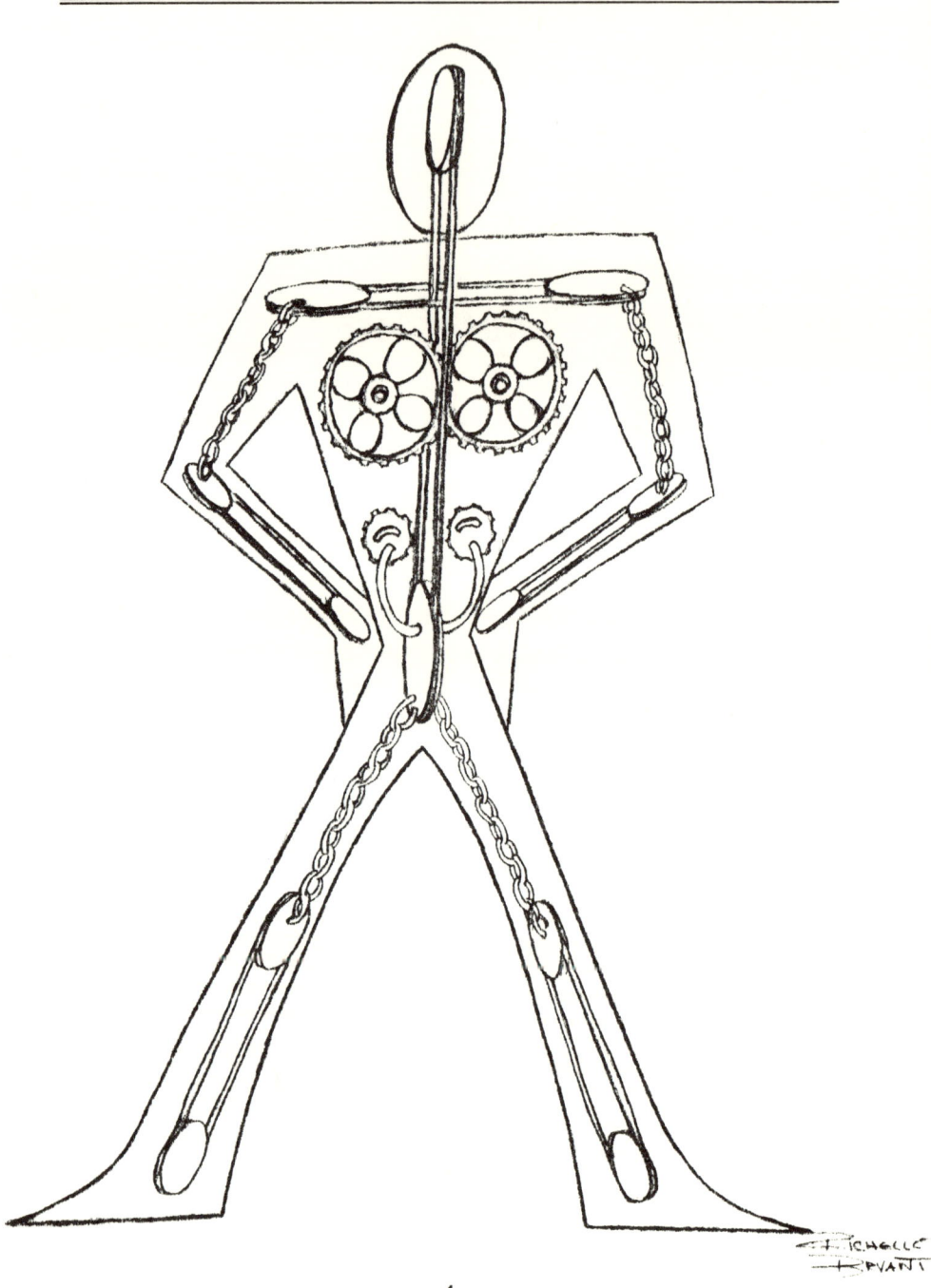

4

body as a sophisticated piece of machinery responding only to machine-like programming, and of disease or illness as an invasion of the natural system--that led to the current methods of health care. These methods, I might add, generally have nothing to do with maintaining wellness but rather are aimed at treating **disease**, and there is a significant difference between these two approaches. Nevertheless, of importance here, is the point that mind "stuff" and body "stuff" have traditionally been viewed as different "stuffs," and, further, that the body-brain was mechanical, somehow like a machine, and it has been treated that way by medicine for the past few hundred years.

As the idea of a separate mind and body developed, there was no room, with few exceptions, for such matters as thought processes. Religious healings, placebo effects, techniques of curing the self using the power of the mind, were ignored or relegated to matters of the clergy. Such happenings were not worth investigating, and besides, they did not occur with "normal" people under controlled circumstances. Only fanatics of one kind or another, such as faith healers or psychic surgeons, continued the search for an understanding of these phenomena in an effort to use the results.

Today, most people believe that to stay healthy you need to keep fit, exercise, avoid "catching" any germs, and more importantly, be lucky. Some others believe that health is a genetic characteristic and that you have to live with what you inherited from your parents. A few are aware that certain types of behavior can influence the type of disease you may experience--for example, the executive who suffers from ulcers. There is, however, a small minority who believe that there is a connection between expectation, thought processes and good health. For this minority, health could be a matter of one's belief system and coping strategy.

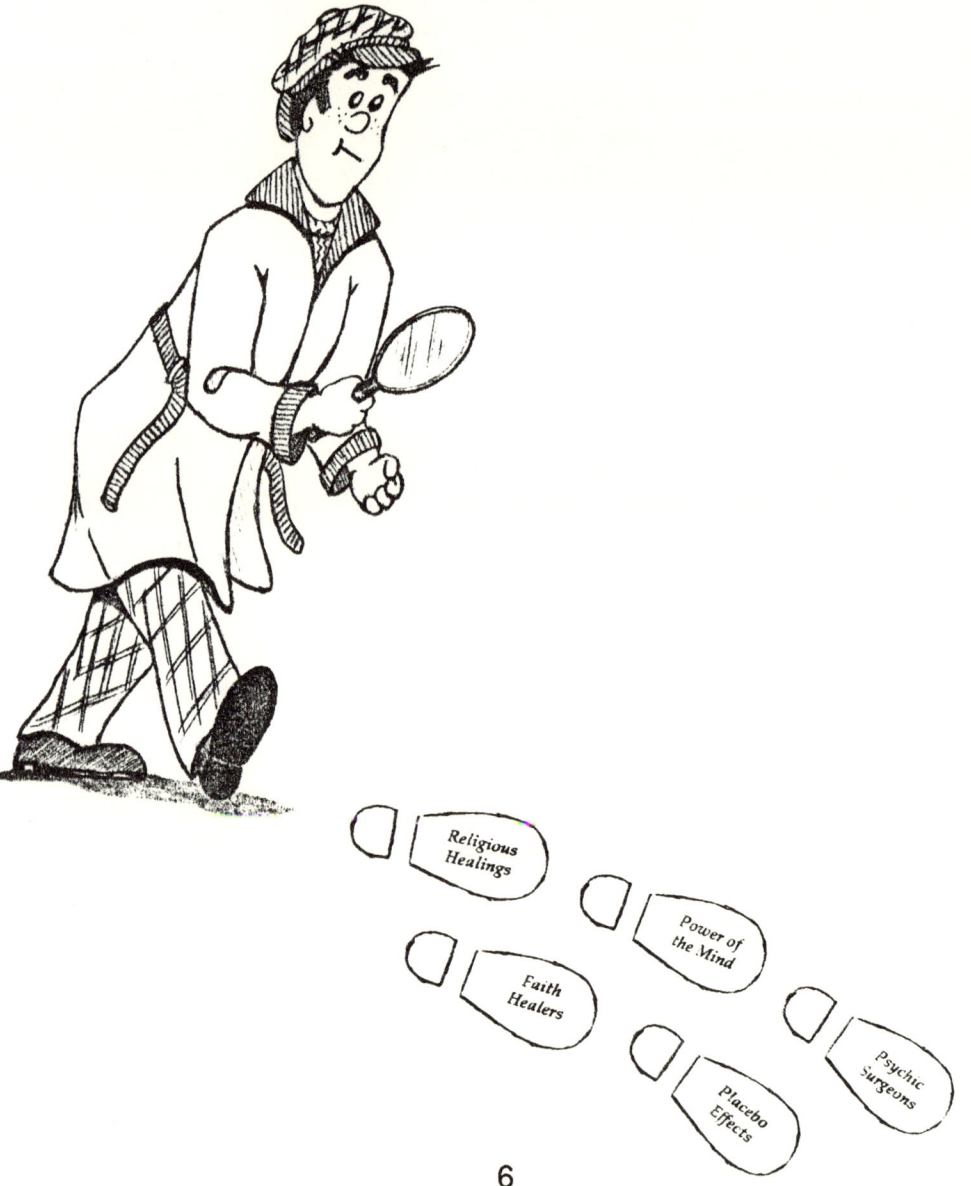

Religious Healings

Power of the Mind

Faith Healers

Placebo Effects

Psychic Surgeons

Chapter Three

My Story

Most of us learn best through our own experiences. For me, an important clue regarding the power of the mind over health occurred when I was a child. This is my story:

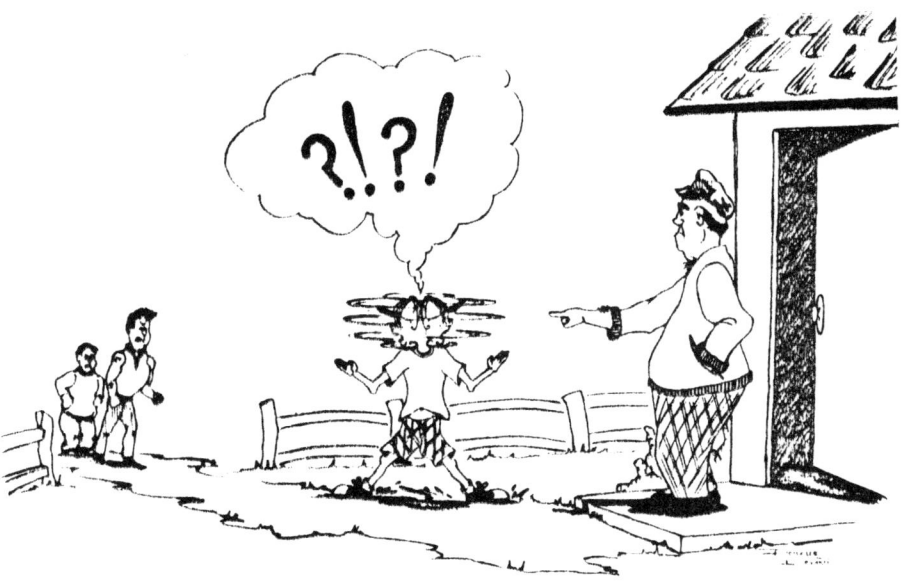

When I was very young, two older boys chased me home from school. My father was upset and promised to "whip" me if I ran away again. I didn't want to go to school the next day. Panic set in. Alas, I didn't have to. The next morning I was ill. Days later, the physician diagnosed rheumatic fever. The physician told my parents and me what to expect as the disease progressed and that is pretty much what happened...at least for a while. After a year and a half, I distinctly remember deciding not to be ill. It was time to go out and play---to ride a bicycle---to say hello to my first crush, to shoot marbles, and so forth. I decided to get well, and almost overnight I was well.

It is a popular misconception that tough guys pick on the weaker individuals who cannot fight back. Most of the tough guys I know will pick a fight with the "leader of the pack" just to prove their superiority. So, when I went back to school, the tough guys did not bother me anymore for I was a poor skinny kid who had been ill with a mysterious disease for more than a year and a half.

Time passed, and soon I was growing by leaps and bounds, reaching almost my full height very early. My father, who carried a gun for some fifty years because he spent his entire life either in the military or in some form of law enforcement, had no patience for a sissy of a boy whose name was the same as his. He paid for a health club where I learned self-defonse. By the time I was in the sixth grade, all those tough kids wanted to bully or fight me again. Pretty soon I was fighting very frequently. Then I found myself in a no-win situation, for suddenly my father spoke to me as if I were scum--trouble waiting to happen, always fighting. I had thought he wanted me to be tough, but my ability to fight was rewarded with acts or words of condemnation. I was confused. First my father had told me never to run from anyone and that if I did he would beat me, and then he treated me as though I were a juvenile delinquent for not running!

I am sure that my father was equally confused--or perhaps I just never understood him. I am certain that he did not intend to place me in that situation. However, the aim of this story is not to place blame on anyone, but to show you the choices I made.

As children we all have a need to please our parents. Suddenly I had a relapse of rheumatic fever. I distinctly remember being aware that I was no longer a threat to anyone, in fact, many of the kids who would have been possible threats to me formerly, felt sympathy for me instead. At that time it did not occur to me that there was a connection between my becoming ill and the **need** I had to avoid conflict. While I was sick I did not have to work out how to please my father, whether by fighting or by running away. This sudden relapse occurred when I was in my teens, at my fittest, involved in sports, scouting, and other outdoor activities. No physical warning--just a relapse. The heart murmur that my mother said I had after the first bout with the disease suddenly returned. For all intents and purposes, the disease took me back, or rather I should say, I took myself back to the circumstances where my parents had lavished me with care and attention and the outside world held no threat to me.

Fortunately for me it was not long before this subconscious strategy again failed to produce the desired result. I say fortunate because I could well have never recovered entirely. Once again, when I said I had had enough of being ill, I regained my good health. I wanted to enjoy life, and at that point athletics were important to me. Then, one night after a basketball game in which I had played all four quarters without substitution, the coach arranged for physicals. I was nervous. If I did not pass the physical, I would not be allowed to continue playing. Somewhat to my surprise, not only did I not have a heart murmur or any other difficulties but one of my friends who seemed fit as the proverbial fiddle, was diagnosed with high blood pressure. He was benched--but not me!

Years later a physician friend of mine examined me in a routine physical. No heart murmur. When I told him of the history of rheumatic fever he explained that back in the fifties physicians had often misdiagnosed many diseases as rheumatic fever. That was the answer--total and complete.

Years passed, and one day I fell prey to the usual seasonal influenza. At home, ill, pampering myself, I received a phone call that required immediate attention. I decided to exert a little "mind over matter" and make myself well. By the time I had traveled across town, most of the symptoms were gone. Suddenly, I began to realize that perhaps I was taking some active part in the choice of what disease I might contract and when and where I might contract it.

At this time in my life I was interested in eastern metaphysics, and I kept coming across the idea that we had the ability to heal ourselves. I reasoned that if you could make yourself well, you must also be able to make yourself ill--even if it was somehow done unconsciously. Was this really possible? If so, how? I searched the library. There were hundreds of stories, just like the one I have shared with you about my own health, and vast volumes of historical information about a time in history when there were many Asclepiad healing centers and people were cured with drama, humor, physical exercise, and dreams! These Asclepiad healing centers began with the ancient Greeks and spread throughout most of our western civilizations. And of course there were very many stories, too many to count, from religious persons of every faith who had experienced seemingly miraculous cures. Surprisingly, at least to me, there were also a number of scientific papers, articles and books that also suggested a mind-body connection. I began to wonder if the popular views on disease were really true. What if disease was not something you "caught" but was sometimes a behavioral strategy? There was certainly enough evidence from my own life to support such a theory.

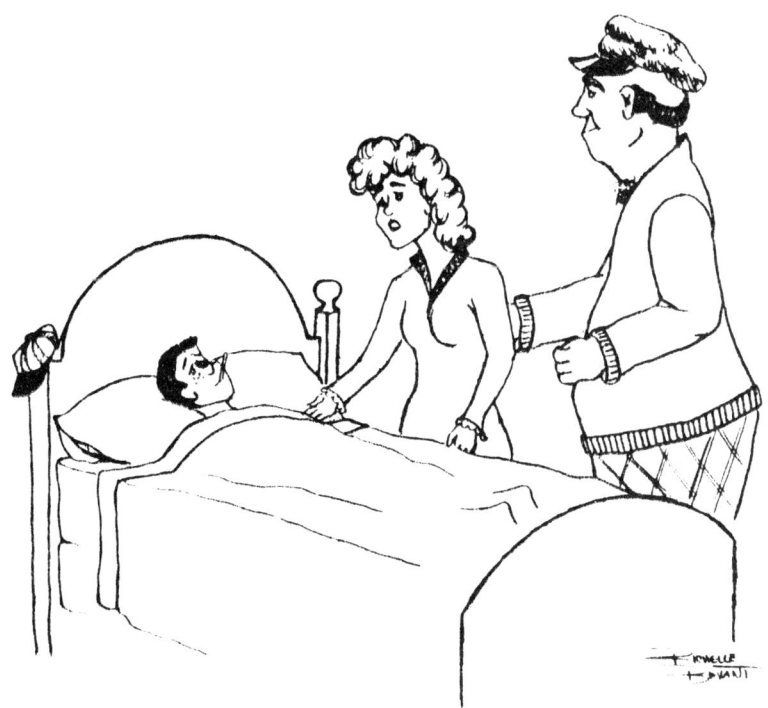

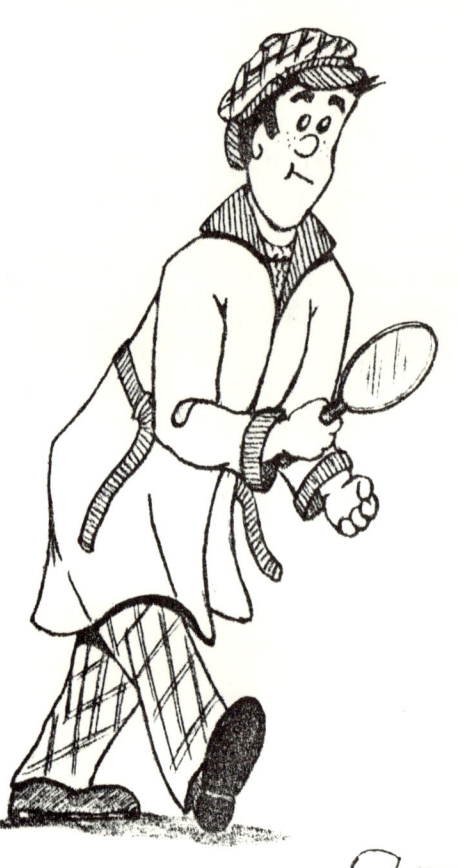

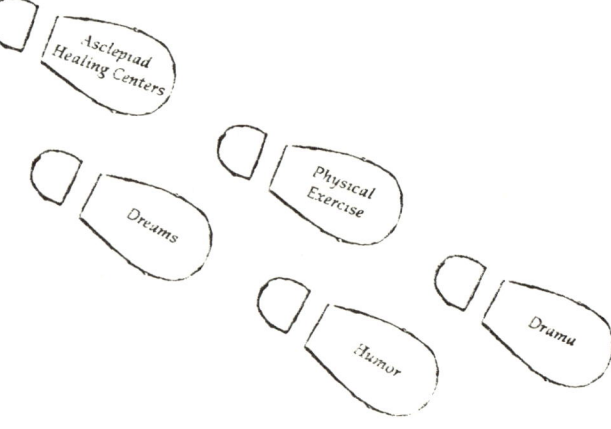

Asclepiad Healing Centers

Dreams

Physical Exercise

Humor

Drama

Chapter Four

A Two-Way Communication?

Most of us are aware of, even if we have not ourselves witnessed, certain forms of hypnotic phenomena that defy traditional definition. One such unforgettable phenomenon I witnessed was performed by the late Professor Carl Leprecht. While teaching a course to lie-detection examiners, he placed himself in wide-eyed hypnosis. On cue his body became rigid, and two officers picked him up and suspended him between two chairs. His head rested at mid-skull on one chair, and his ankles rested on the other. A complete body catalepsy, and he continued to lecture! If I had not seen this with my own eyes, I would have doubted nearly anyone who might have told me the story. But there, in front of approximately thirty law enforcement people, was Leprecht doing things with his body that defied possibility; but how can anything defy possibility and still be possible? How could simple words or thoughts turn the human body into a rigid bar? Further, how could the cells of the body process these messages?

One of the pioneers in lie detection was Cleve Baxter. He demonstrated that plants not only are sensitive to their surroundings but can literally identify an individual. This

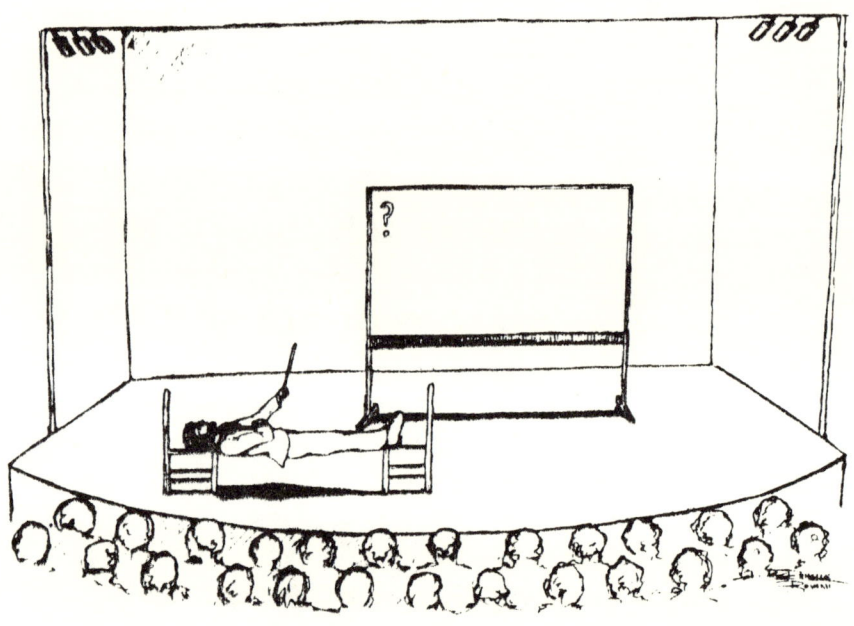

phenomenon challenges many of our ideas about consciousness.

While speaking at the Ohio Academy I met a fellow presenter who had taken some of Baxter's work a step further. Dr. Bruce Lipton is a researcher and teacher at Stanford School of Medicine. For years his specialty was cellular biology. Bruce told me of an experiment where cells of the body were removed and transported to distances as much as five miles away from the host organ, or person. Both were closely monitored. When one was traumatized, the other responded sympathetically regardless of the distance. Conversely, when the cells were traumatized, the body responded. In other words, one of your cells five miles away from you, will respond immediately when you are hurt! Somehow the distance does not separate the cell from the larger body of cells from which it was removed.

Is this an example of cell consciousness? If it is, is it possible for the cell to cause behavior? That is, could the cells of the body actually provide the impetus for behavior in contrast to the classic belief where behavior originates in the brain and the body just goes along with whatever the brain decides? Could there be a two-way system? That sometimes both operate to produce behavior? That they even cooperate? The cells cooperating with the brain to produce an illness or disease that meets some need of the "stuff" we call consciousness or mind? Again, going back to the story of when I was a child, the cells of my body were certainly being very *cooperative* when they developed an illness, thus giving my *mind* an alternative to having to face a situation it could not (or did not want to) handle. The questions remain. Does the mind have a role in dis-ease and does the body imitate the mind's expectation? Further, can we even ask these questions as though we might get answers or be able to do something about what we find?

The investigator in me decided to go back a little further into the recent history of the mind's role in wellness to see if I could uncover some more clues.

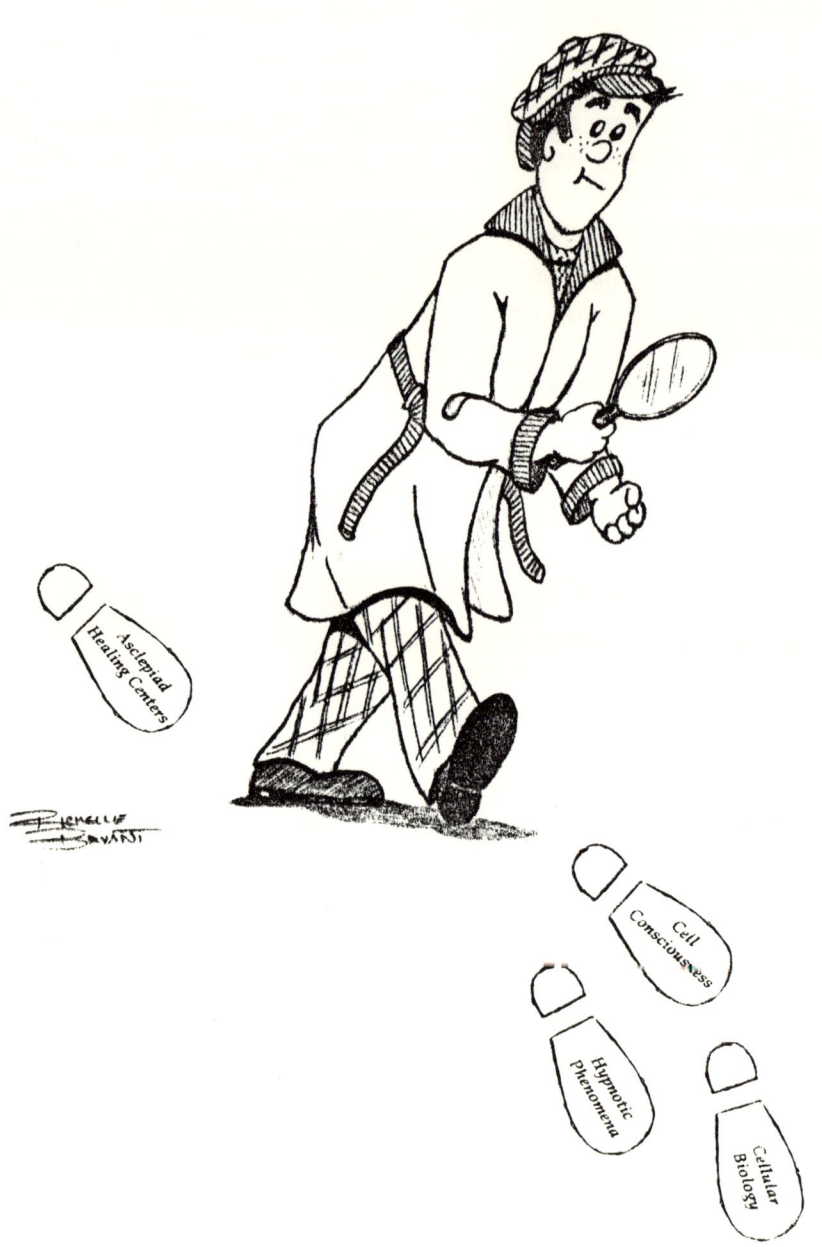

Chapter Five

Some Interesting Phenomena

In 1765 Franz Anton Mesmer used magnets to produce miraculous cures. Later it was said by most critics that the results Mesmer obtained were due to the power of suggestion or hypnosis. One single idea, on its own, could produce the phenomenon demonstrated by Mesmer, or so some argued. There were also those who used imagination and imitation to produce an altered state of consciousness, and so healed the blind and the terminally ill.

It is amazing how ideas change over time. With recent developments in technology, we are not far from believing that it may have been the influence of hypnosis, imagination, imitation, **and** the magnets that worked the miracles of Mesmer's time. For years Mesmer and his followers cured patients of a large number of different illnesses. In time Mesmer was disgraced, and he died in obscurity. The disgrace was due in part to the scientific community's inability to understand Mesmer's work. The magnets alone did not cure; nevertheless, **something** did. Mesmer may have had his theories wrong, but the ill who had been cured remained for the most part cured. Why was this fact overlooked? Mesmer was politically unpopular, but that was unimportant to those he treated and cured. Of course, other factors were involved here, but the fact remains that something totally out of the ordinary process of mechanical medicine was at work. Words that could heal?

In the 1880s, Jean Martin Charcot regularly demonstrated one of his favorite hypnotic procedures to medical personnel at the Salpetriere hospital in France. Under hypnosis, a patient suffering from hysterical paralysis (paralysis for which there is no physical cause) would stand and walk on Charcot's command. Out of hypnosis the same person would "crumple to the ground." Were the hypnotic suggestions causing the cells to remember, and thus causing a change in physiology, or wellness? Were they removing the psychological barriers that caused the dysfunction in the first place? Freud theorized before the end of his career that "emotions not expressed in words or actions would find expression in some sort of physical ailment." Did the words used in hypnosis alter the emotion?

Now wait a minute. How can the mind, or memory, or emotion play such a significant role in curative powers? And if this is real, why hasn't it been exhaustively studied by science?

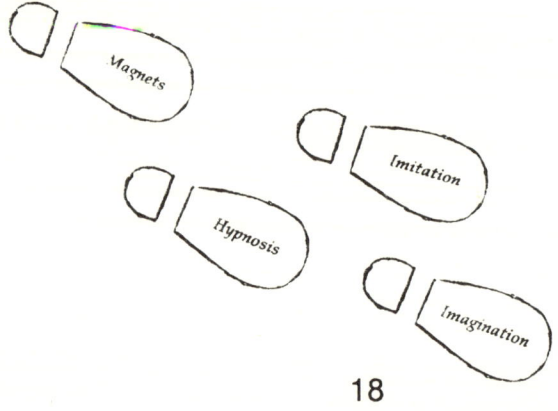

Chapter Six

Personality

Many health care professionals tend to treat personality in physical wellness issues as though it were always constant, but if there are no variations, what accounts for "normal" personalities and "pathological" personalities? It is important to understand that there are indeed great variations in personality before we can understand the human condition. In fact, personality is a feature that is not unique to humans, for we all know that animals each have their own personalities. Does personality have anything to do with illness?

I asked these questions. To the library I ventured, but instead of discovering a scarcity of evidence I found that the literature bulged with experiments and observations showing clearly that personality does have a connection with illness. In fact, the "seven psychosomatic ailments"--peptic ulcers, ulcerative colitis, hypertension, hyperthyroidism, rheumatoid arthritis, neurodermatitis, and asthma are thought to occur mainly in certain personality types. One of the most convincing evidences that personality contributes to body processes were the reports of multiple personality patients. One personality may be totally normal in every physiological sense, and yet with the sudden shift of personalities, some as quick as the snap of a finger, the second personality may be hypoglycemic. Blood chemistry altering in seconds? How does a personality shift alter body chemistry in seconds? Other such patients have demonstrated everything from eye color change to having one menstruation cycle per month for every personality within the patient.

A personal belief system, such as personality, capable of causing an instant change in the way the cells behave? What mechanism allows for such a sudden and dramatic shift in the person's blood chemistry? What "trigger" makes that possible?

I looked further and found that herpes has been linked to loneliness; positive mood, hope, and social support was linked to cancer survival; tough mindedness and a will to live with survival of AIDS. Could that all be true?

Madeline Visintaines of the University of Pennsylvania linked helplessness to cancer. She concluded that helplessness is somehow interpreted by the body as an absence of "the ability of the organism to resist tumor development."

Researchers at Duke University showed hostility and mistrust to be key predictors of heart disease and early death. H. J. Eysenck summarized a group of European studies and found the following:

1.   "Individuals who tended to repress their emotions in the face of stress were far likelier than others to die of cancer."

2.   "Those who rated high on emotional frustration and

aggression had a high rate of cardiac related deaths."

3.   "Personality variables were more predictive than smoking in the occurrence of lung cancer. For example, smoking was virtually a pre-requisite for getting lung cancer, but of the smokers, only the emotionally repressive types seemed to contract the disease."

I looked further. Personality was tied to literally clusters of diseases. At Georgia State University, researchers discovered that people with eating and drinking disorders frequently suffered from depression, indecision, chronic fatigue, low self-esteem, physical weakness, and hopelessness. At the University of Texas at Austin, higher cancer rates in mice were linked to blocked emotional expressiveness and under-stimulation.

Karl Goodkin of Stanford University School of Medicine believes, from the evidence of studies of women prone to cancer, that the usual cancer personality is;
1.   overly cooperative,
2.   extremely self-sacrificing,
3.   overly optimistic to the extent of being in denial of reality, and
4.   sociable to a fault.
In contrast, however, women who developed **cervical** cancer were characterized as;
1.   hostile,
2.   quite fearless,
3.   unusually hard-headed,
4.   punitive toward others, and
5.   very blunt in social situations.

But wait a minute. What are we discovering from all these personality models, which seem to contradict each other? A quick review reveals a similarity in the description "extreme"-- **extreme** self-sacrifice, **extreme** bluntness, and so forth.

I quickly learned that personality profile characteristics have been developed for many illnesses besides cancer. Personality could indeed one day become a significant means of predicting which illnesses an individual could suffer from. Emotional states such as grief have been shown to lower the immune response, and positive emotions have been shown to improve the immune response. In fact, epinephrine and norepinephrine, which act to turn up or down the immune system, have repeatedly been shown to be linked to mood states. For example, Dr. Ziad Kronfol found that the immune systems in depressed patients were less responsive than those of normal individuals, and he believes that is due to stress hormones in the body.

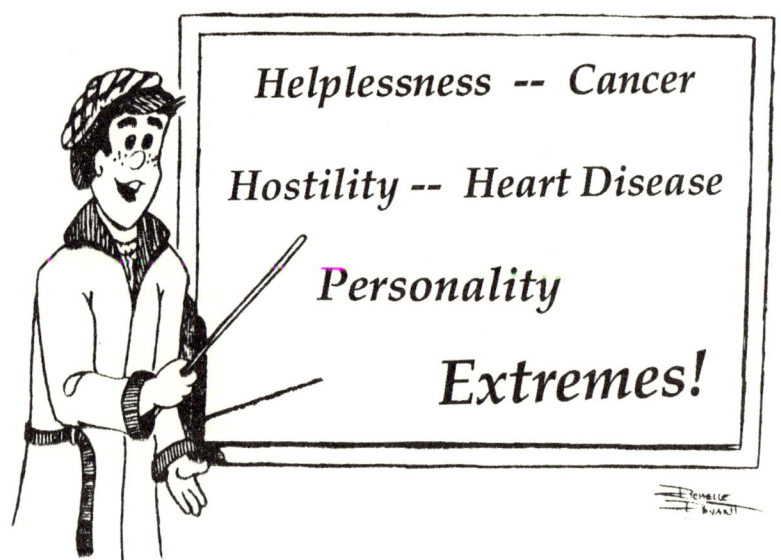

22

Chapter Seven

Stress

Satisfied that I was not going in circles, I continued to pore over the literature. Stress as a factor in disease began to appear more and more frequently. But what is stress? Is conflict stress? What about the kind of conflict that arises as a result of choice? Is indecision a stressful matter? What role does mind play in stress?

An Ohio State University researcher reported that marital discontent weakened the immune response. George Soloman of UCLA reported that the stress and strain of life crises diminished the immune response.

Ted Melnechuk, director of research communications for the Institute For The Advancement Of Health adds the following observation:

1. Men married to dying women have a lowered immune response.

2. Monkeys separated from their mothers experience immune suppression.

3. Visual imagery has been shown to decrease tumor growth.

4. Nerve cells have been shown to travel from the brain to the thymus and back to the brain demonstrating a two way communication with this important relay station for immune substances.

It was time for me to apply some of this information. In 1988 and 1989 Dr. Robert Youngblood, a cosmetic surgeon, used a subliminal audio cassette I created for reducing stress and anxiety in patients about to undergo surgical operations. He examined the records of the 360 previous patients who had undergone the same or similar surgical operations to determine the average anesthetic requirements. We reasoned that lowering patient stress, anxiety, and other related feelings would result in lowering anesthetic requirements. We were right. The audio cassette was used before, during, and after surgery. The overall anesthetic requirement was lowered by 32% in the patient group that received the subliminal tape as compared with the 360 previous patients who had not been exposed to the subliminal tape. Interestingly enough, post-secondary care was also substantially reduced.

Hypnosis, as we have seen, has been shown to be effective in matters of health. In fact, it has been demonstrated effective in the care or treatment of asthma, hypertension, bleeding, dermatitis, and various emotional states, in speeding the rate of healing, as an aid to breast enlargement, and much more. In fact, one of the studies I participated in was at a medical facility in Nevada. This facility offers a number of different "high tech" medical testing procedures, including magnetic resonance imaging, or MRI. This procedure is

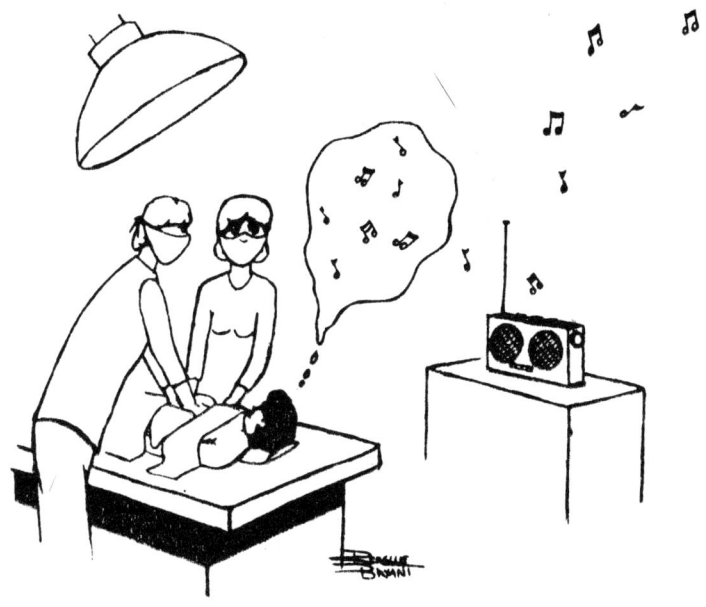

designed to look at soft tissue and requires that one be "loaded down a skid into a chamber," to use the words of one of the technicians, that is very small in diameter. One problem they frequently came across was emotional stress and a fear of confined places. Another problem they often had to deal with was relative to the anxiety attached to this type of testing. This meant that in some instances, they had to medicate a patient even for the less frightening CAT scan.

The medical facility asked us to create an audio program that would help these conditions. We used a combination of special frequencies for altering brain wave activity while stimulating certain effects and added subliminal messages and guided imagery or hypnosis. The results were significant. According to a senior technician, patient refusals to undergo the testing were completely eliminated when the tape was used.

In 1991, Sheldon Cohen of Carnegie Mellon University in Pittsburgh reported a study that links emotional stress to the common cold. Cohen's group found that the rates of respiratory infection and colds were directly related to stress levels, even when allowances were made for various influences on the immune system such as age, sex, education, allergies, weight, viral status prior to the study, cigarette and alcohol use, exercise, diet, quality of sleep, number of housemates, and the number of times the housemates suffered from infections. The relationship between stress and colds was also shown not to be affected by personality types. Could it really be that the common cold is stress-related?

Candace Pert, chief of brain biochemistry for the National Institute of Mental Health, suggests that "emotions are the key to health." In fact, she and her colleague Michael Ruff have been working with Peptide T, one of the messenger molecules in the body that apparently converts emotions into biological happenings. Drs. Pert and Ruff have found that this substance can help alleviate AIDS symptoms, stop the spread of the HIV virus and, in some cases, even neutralize its toxicity. Dr. Pert also asserts that "the same chemicals that control mood in the brain control tissue integrity of the body." Many of the messenger molecules which are associated with emotion have been discovered to be strategically located throughout the body. Brain chemicals centered in the body? One of these molecules, CCK, forms a lining from the esophagus throughout the intestines and, according to Pert, may "explain why some people talk about **gut feelings**". Additionally, and all-important as a clue, Pert insists that placebo analgesia, analgesia triggered by suggestion, is an altered state dependent on messenger molecules.

Sorting through all the data, doing my own research, I continued to add new clues.

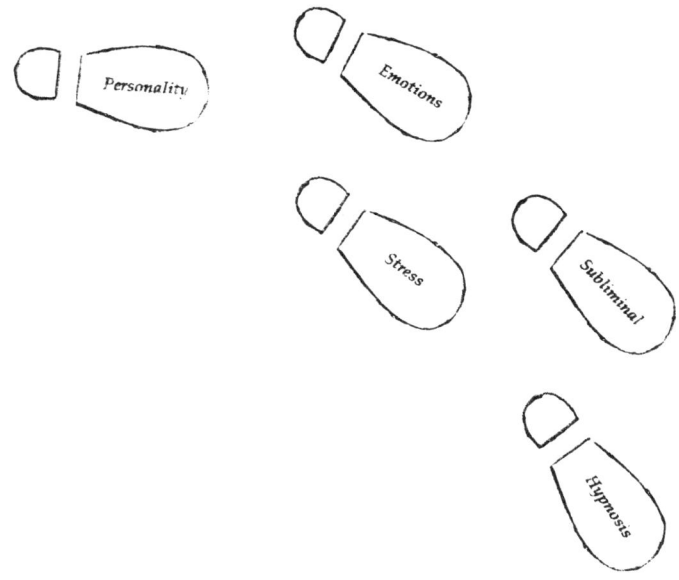

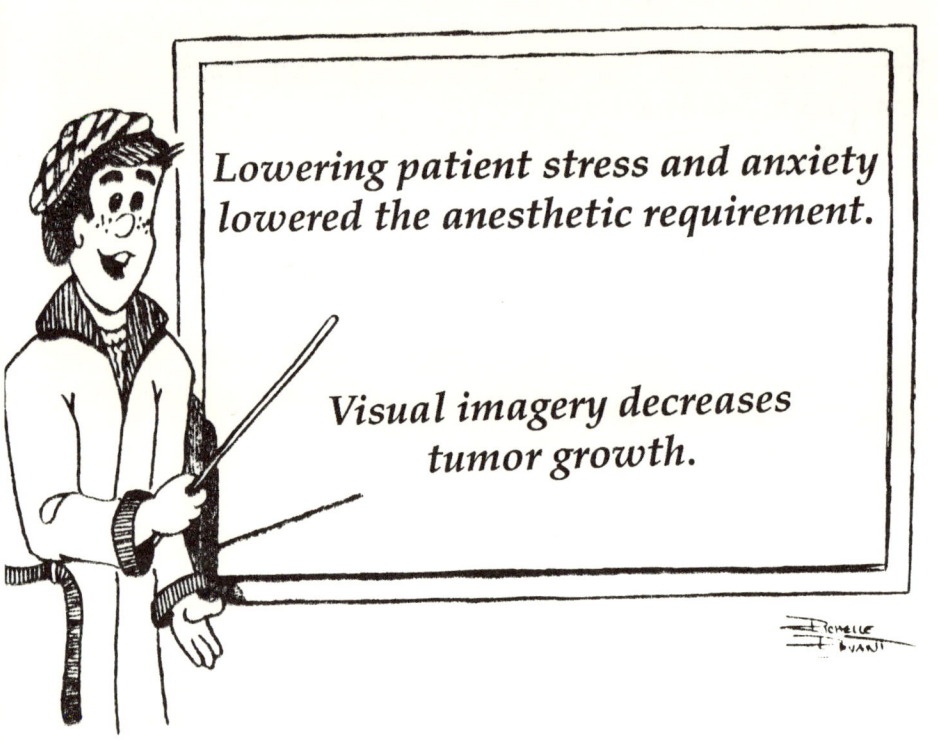

28

Chapter Eight

Conditioning

Most people have heard of Pavlov's dogs and know that they were trained to salivate at the sound of a bell. This occurred because the dogs were delivered food whenever a bell was rung. Over time, with sufficient repetitions, the dogs came to expect food **whenever** they heard the bell. This is known as classical conditioning. In the mid-1970s Robert Ader conducted some classical Pavlovian conditioning with rats, trying to train them to dislike saccharin-flavored water. After the animals drank the water, Ader injected them with a drug which made the rats nauseated. During the experiment many of the rats died. That was totally unexpected but, after careful review, Ader discovered that the drug was a powerful immunosuppressant, that is, it prevented the immune system from functioning. Was it possible that while Ader was conditioning his rats to dislike saccharin that he had accidentally conditioned their immune system? Was it possible to condition the immune system to stop working? Ader decided yes and later discovered that two Soviet scientists had conditioned a guinea pig "to release antibodies when they scratched its skin." Classical conditioning of the immune system? Is it possible that we may have

29

"conditioned" responses to certain diseases? Could a person's expectation actually be the conditioning mechanism?

Could it be that one of the reasons many of us do not experience miraculous healing, extended life spans and good health is due to some conditioning, some other enculturation. Does the television condition us to expect a cold's season? Do we learn to be ill? Although we know the pathogens that "cause" illness are "real," does the individual have the ultimate control as to how the body will respond? If so, how? And after all, to what extent?

Psychologist Ernest Rossi's research convinced him that "human beings cannot always rely on nature to reinstate health because certain short-term responses can become habitual and pathological." Habituation is surely an outward manifestation of expectation. Also, Rossi believes that certain mental events can become imprinted in the body as disease and chronic conditions--memorized, if you will. Originally, this "learned-state" helped us cope with a particular situation, Rossi theorizes. Later, when similar situations occur, we react the way we did the first time, even though there is no longer a "need." For example, to avoid a particular situation, an individual becomes ill. Rather than relate the illness to the need to avoid a situation, however, the individual could relate it to the time of year, a certain food, a particular fragrance, etc. The seasonal cold a person experiences may therefore be due more to a memory triggering off the illness than to the change in external temperature. This process of "state-dependent learning," or responding as a result of a state or condition, is bounded by amnesia, which is simply to say that we are no longer consciously aware of it.

How can we undo this conditioning? Are we any closer to solving the mystery?

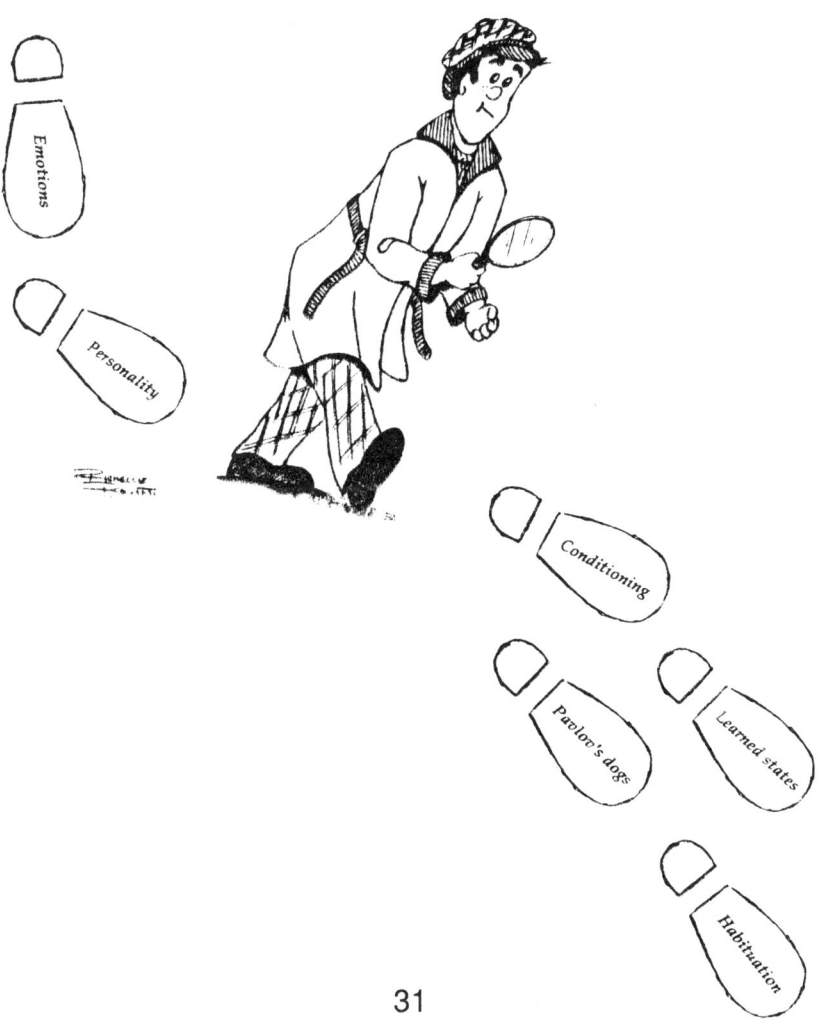

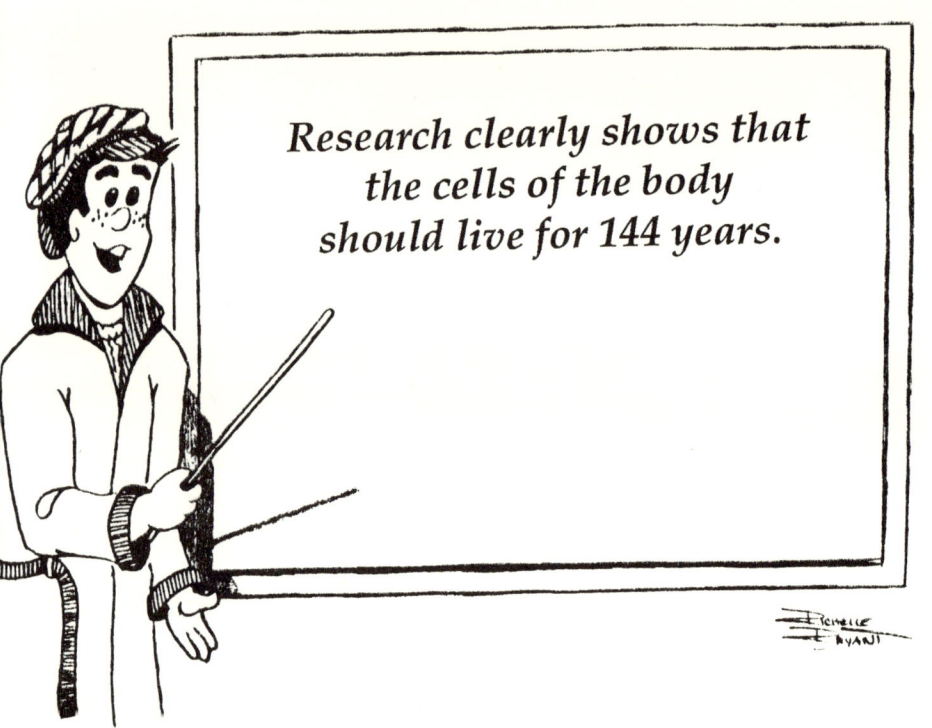

Chapter Nine

What We Expect Is What We Get

In 1990, I attended the annual SKY Foundation's convention in Philadelphia, Pennsylvania, where I met a fellow presenter, Dr. Joel Posner, who was speaking on the subject of yoga and longevity. Dr. Posner, a professor of physiology, stated that research clearly shows that the cells of the body should live for 144 years. The body should therefore not die for at least 144 years unless the mind somehow interferes with the natural pattern of the cell.

Research has also clearly shown that when subjects in their seventies exercise at the same minimal level as subjects in their twenties, the muscle mass generation (growth) is the same for both groups. This supports the old saying, "Use it or lose it." But what conditions us to accept age as being the decay of the body? And what can be done to un-condition this learning? What experiences, including expectation or attitude, cause us to alter the natural cellular programming (life expectancy)? Why is it that we are so familiar with some of the answers related to diet, sunlight, drugs, and so on and yet still so in the dark about the essential mental contributors to good health and long life? Or are we?

Many traditional and historical myths cause us to believe in the idea of miraculous healing. The stories speak of a time when men lived to be hundreds of years old, of a time when everyone **expected** to be well. Is that it? Is it possible that the myth of disease has replaced the myth of wellness? Do most of us expect to get sick, become ill, and then die at some point in our lives? Is this a form of the self-fulfilling prophecy that reduces our time here on earth to a fraction of the at least 144 years the cell is expected to maintain perfect life? How many of us expect to be sick as a normal course of events in our lives? How many of us expect to be ill each year? How many of us expect to live to the age of 144? How much of an investment do each of us and our society at large have in the "illness" paradigm? Is it possible to be well all of your life---for whatever period of time that may naturally be? Is it even responsible to suggest such an idea? What would happen if all of us suddenly changed our beliefs, energies, and other investments entirely, so that we **expected** to be well? Is that an irresponsible question?

It is fun to imagine a world where there are no television commercials selling remedies for the dreaded annual illnesses and other maladies. No more constipation commercials. No more hemorrhoid commercials. No more television, or radio, or print media, or conversation about preparing for illness, physical and mental disabilities, and so forth as we grow older. What would it be like if we didn't have a world of afflictions to discuss, think about, or otherwise invest our energies in? Does all of that really even matter? Is it relevant to health and wellness? Truly relevant?

The Sufis have a story about time and pomegranates that may shed a little anecdotal light on our questions: Once upon a time, in a land far away, there was a young man who wanted to become a healer. He knew of a legendary healer under whom he wished to train. He therefore set out on a journey to find the healer and learn the secrets of his practice and ways.

After a long and trying period he finally found the healer and without hesitation went up to him. The healer saw that the boy was sincere and decided to take him on as a student.

After weeks of training, the two were sitting on the porch of the healer's modest home one day when a stranger approached from the distance. He was crumpled over and moved in an odd and peculiar way.

The healer said to his student, "See that man coming up the path--what he needs is pomegranates." The young man watched as the healer listened to the patient tell an agonizing tale of woeful experiences with his affliction, including the struggle he had gone through just to make the journey to the healer's doorstep. Finally, the healer put his hand on the patient's shoulder and spoke softly. "Yes, I can see you have suffered. I can see you are ready to leave your illness behind. My friend, I am certain that your disease is due to a shortage of a particular substance available in high concentrations in pomegranates. Eat three pomegranates a day for the next week and your health will return."

The patient left and within a couple of weeks returned standing erect with a basket of food for the healer and the blessings of a deeply grateful self and family.

A short time later another stranger came down the road to the healer's home. He also walked in the same odd and peculiar way and was all bent over as he approached. The student noticed the stranger and excitedly said, "What he needs is pomegranates." The healer nodded in agreement without really looking up from his porch chair. The student then pleaded with the healer to allow him to treat the patient. Finally the healer agreed, and the student went out to meet the patient and tell him of his cure. Approaching the man, the student blurted out, "What you need is pomegranates!" The stranger stopped. He looked at the student and said, "I came all this way for this non-sense! Pomegranates---rubbish! Some healer you are," and he turned and went away.

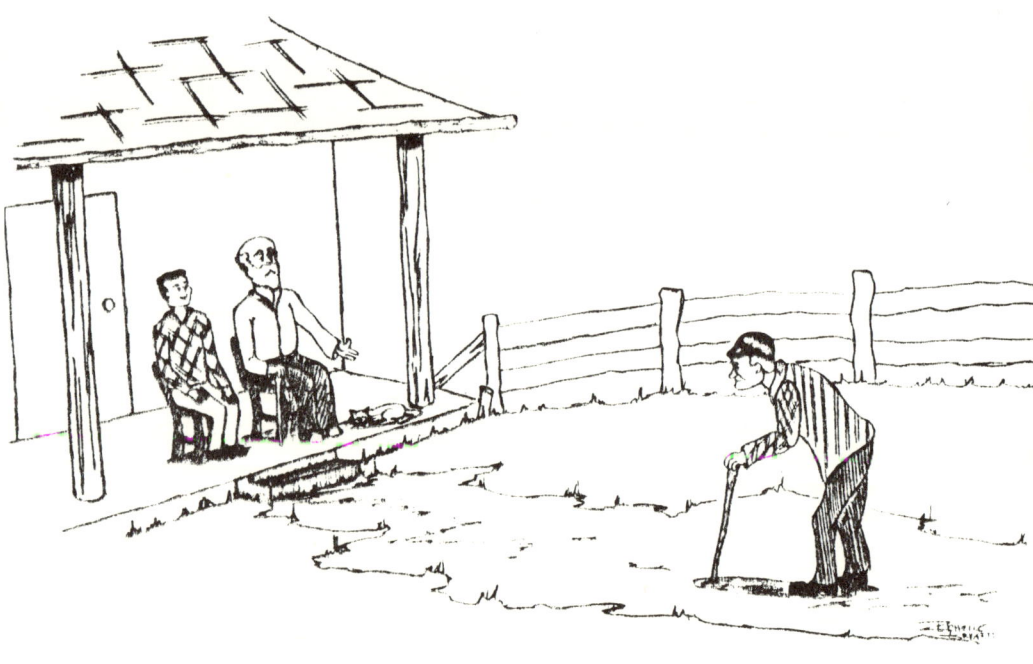

One aspect to this story has to do with the expectation of the patient. Another is that the student did not understand the necessity of **time** and pomegranates. The afflicted person's expectation of the great healer and his ability to tell of his suffering and finally find relief were entirely overlooked by the student. The student had taken only a mechanical learning from the healer and assumed that pomegranates alone would cure. For that reason, both the student healer and the patient were disappointed in the end.

In the spring of 1991 I conducted a survey among physicians who had consented to their patients using a special experimental subliminal program for cancer remission. The aim of the study was to look at life expectancy in comparison with the actual mortality rates of patients with cancer who used the subliminal program. The questionnaire went to physicians whose patients had received the subliminal program two to four years earlier. The twelve questions were rated on a scale of 1 to 5:
    1. strongly disagree,
    2. disagree,
    3. neutral,
    4. agree, and
    5. strongly agree.

The twelve questions consisted of four general categories:
    1. the patient's attitude toward their disease before they used the program,
    2. the patient's attitude toward their disease after they used the program,
    3. the patient's survival and quality of life, and
    4. how the physician felt about the patient's believing health could be affected by the patient's mind.

This survey revealed many interesting findings including significant remission rates, for 38% of the so-called terminal patients are in remission at the time of this writing. One other interesting and overwhelmingly obvious result was found that may surprise you. Of the four subcategories, which do you think would be the most consistent factor affecting the life expectancy or remission rate in the patient?

Most people believe that it is the patient's attitude, even though those same people would say that a terminal disease such as cancer cannot be affected just by changing the patient's attitude. It wasn't the patient's attitude, however, but the **physician's** attitude that was the most important factor in determining whether the patient lived or died.

If the physician did not believe that the patient's involvement with the subliminal tape or the patient's attitude could affect the cancer, the patient died, regardless of which treatment procedure was used--radiation, chemotherapy, and so on. The patient died regardless of the patient's own attitude toward the disease or its ultimate outcome. The one factor present in virtually every case was the physician's attitude.

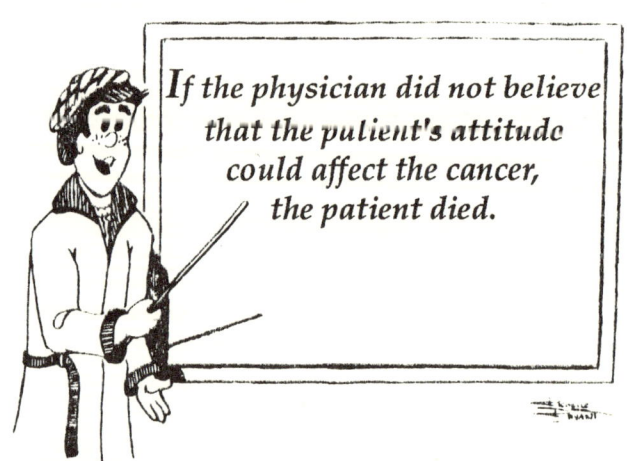

If the physician did not believe that the patient's attitude could affect the cancer, the patient died.

Taking into account only those patients whose physicians agreed, to varying degrees, that the mind played a role in the patient's health, then the survival/remission rate increases to 46%. If we look at those physicians who **strongly** agreed that the mind or attitude of the patient is important to health and/or health care, the survival/remission rate increases to 60%. Narrowing the field still further, where both the patient and the physician tended to believe strongly that the mind played a role in wellness, the rate of survival/remission increased to 100%.

Is it possible that we are being conditioned into ill health by the attitudes of those in authority around us? Is it possible that a physician's sentence of "terminal without hope" is the actual cause of death? Do we rely so totally on the opinion of professionals that we prove them to be correct, even if that means suffering and death? Does the data from our study suggest that the answer to health care is a positive cooperation between the patient and the physician? What is this power of authority about? How do we learn to imitate or act so that pleasing an authority is a priority more important than life? Or do we? After all, maybe this was just a fluke finding. Maybe this is just an extension of the well-known placebo effect, only reversed. Still, a placebo works because of our expectation. Is our "inverted" belief the crux of wellness? If emotion, learning, behavior, and personality are all tied up in wellness, then how we learn how and what to believe is crucial.

Our self-talk is indicative of our attitudes. Norman Cousins writes in **The Anatomy of an Illness** that he healed himself of a terminal illness using positive self-talk and laughter. The story of this wonderful man is worth retelling.

Mr. Cousins learned he was terminally ill with cancer. "How could this be," he questioned. He had always been careful with his health. Finally his physician suggested that the illness may have taken a foothold because of the stress and negative emotions in Cousin's life. The answer was obvious to Norman Cousins. If negative feelings could produce dis-ease, then positive emotions would cure the dis-ease. He therefore systematically obtained every funny film available. Old Laurel and Hardy movies and the like had Mr. Cousins laughing away most of every day. It wasn't long, and laughter had healed. Norman Cousins left the hospital to share his experience with everyone.

Dr. Gerald Jampolski states in both of his works, **Love Is Letting Go of Fear** and **Teach Only Love**, that a person's attitude can and does heal. His attitudinal healing center in California has become famous for just this type of healing. In fact, Jampolski points out that patients in incredible pain "forget" their pain when they help another patient in an urgent situation.

My own work has suggested what I have referred to as *"the warm, fuzzy, fully feeling human experience,"* a term used to describe the way all of us feel when we go to the aid of an injured life form. At that moment, we are so aware of the *"warm and fuzzy"* feeling that glows within us that we forget all about ourselves, immersed, if you will, in our concern for another. Not only do we forget about the fear of pain and discomfort when we are in this situation, but the memory lives on in us as being the best that we can ever be. In short, it feels so good, so natural, so *"warm and fuzzy,"* that it is generally the most rewarding part when that activity is viewed in 20/20 hindsight.

Chapter Ten

A Trip Down Memory Lane

One of the clues that kept "popping out" at me may surprise you, and that is the involvement of memory in health and wellness.

A distinguished physician, Dr. Deepak Chopra, believes that memory, as well as the attitude of a person, plays a large part in wellness and spontaneous remission. Dr. Chopra argues in his marvelous book **Quantum Healing** that patients at the edge of despair, struggling for hope, can replace fear and uncertainty with the **memory of health**. As soon as "the memory returns . . . with enough power to last a lifetime," they experience spontaneous regression of their disease.

Then, while reading a biography of Milton Erickson, I came across some evidence that supports this line of thinking. When he was seventeen, Erickson suffered from a bout of polio which left him almost totally paralyzed. One day his family forgot they had left him alone, tied into the rocking chair they had adapted into a primitive potty. The chair had been placed in the middle of the room, which left Erickson looking longingly at the window, wishing he could at least look out at the farm. Suddenly he became aware that the chair had begun to rock slightly. Was that an accident, or had his wishing to be closer to the window actually stimulated some minimal body movement to set the chair rocking?

In the weeks and months that followed, Erickson focused on remembering how to move, how his fingers felt when grasping a pitch fork, how his body moved when he used to climb trees. Slowly, what had started with the "accidental" rocking of his chair became movements he could consciously control.

After eleven months of intensive self-training, Erickson was walking with the aid of crutches.

The evidence for the importance of memory in health and wellness accumulated when a friend of mine brought me an article. He knew that I was scheduled to give a presentation in Israel on Memory-Dependent Wellness and that I had started a research project on remembering youth. The heading of the article was "Reversing the Clock." It described a landmark research project by Dr. Ellen Langer that reversed certain characteristics of aging.

Dr. Langer of Harvard University took "old people" into the country where they were isolated for one week. The older persons were exposed to "photographs, newspapers, radio (music and advertising) and discussions that were strictly limited to topics current twenty years earlier. At the end of the week, the group became younger looking by three years, gained weight, behaved more independently, and could actually hear better." Memory--relived!

The most convincing final piece of evidence for me that proved memory to be the magical key to health and wellness was an article I read in *Mind Brain Bulletin*. The article stated that neuroscientists had confirmed with PET scans that the hippocampus, a specific area in the brain, played a crucial role in memory. To understand the importance of this finding, you need to know that the hippocampus is the area of the brain which, together with the limbic system, modulates the immune system. Therefore, there is a definite hard-wire connection between memory, emotion, expectation, and wellness.

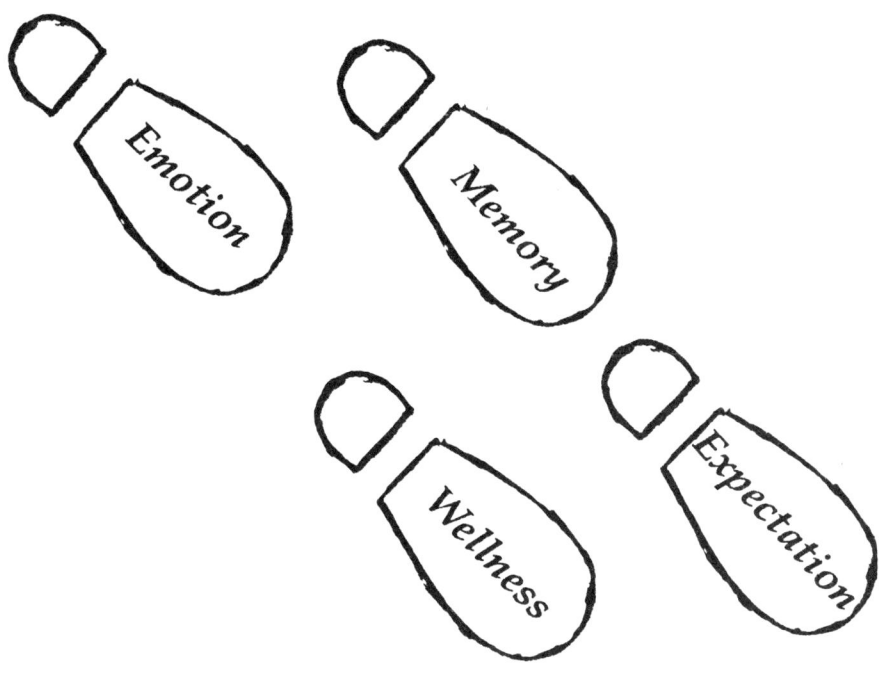

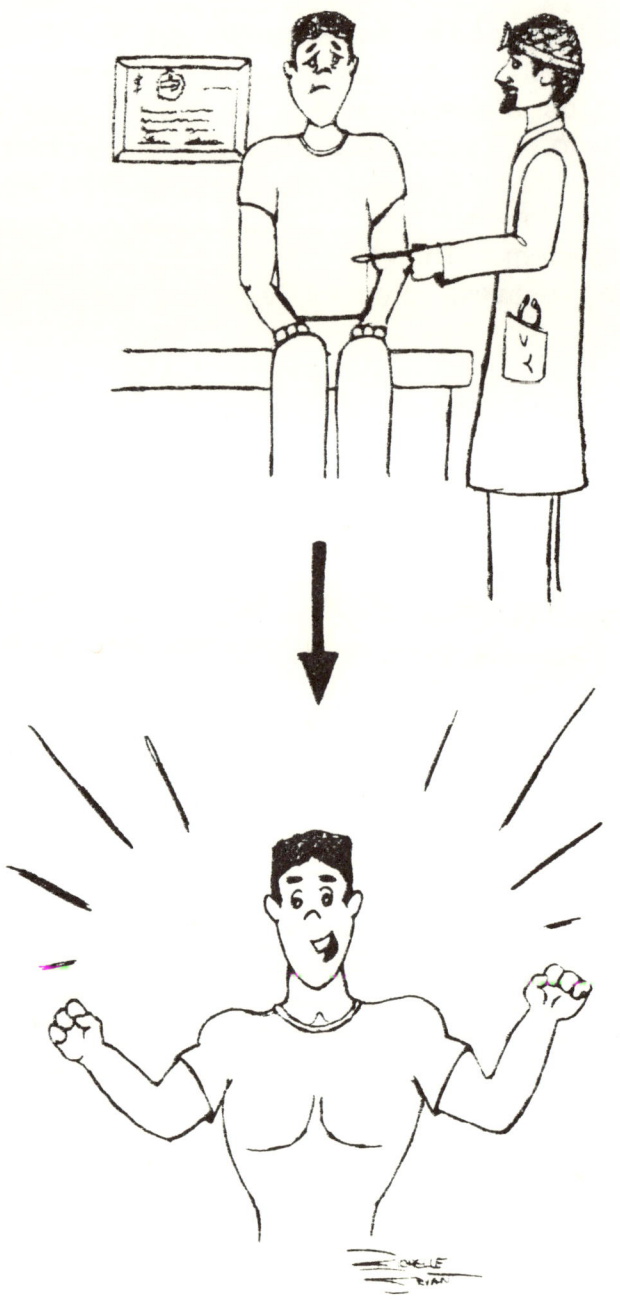

Chapter Eleven

The Power of Belief

So far the clues to the mind's role in wellness and longevity include;

1. the memory of health,
2. positive emotions, and
3. a hopeful versus helpless attitude.

Now we need to look at hope. Everyone knows what helplessness is, but what is hopeful? Not false hope, but good, sound, productive hope. Stories indicate that people who have hope and look at life from the perspective that all will ultimately work out for the best are indeed happier and healthier.

In all the cases of remission, extended good health, miraculous healings, and the like, one thing seems to be present, and that is belief. For some, this is belief in their own higher power: for others, it is an act of knowing wellness will return; for still others, it has been the touch of a healer; and so on; but always, there is **TRUE BELIEF**. Hope is belief.

Belief is not some unchanging this, that, or the other. Belief is dynamic. It is revealed daily in the way we live our life. It can be referred to as active expectation. It is re-enforced over and over again when relied upon each day. It is the one factor each of us can thoroughly instill in ourselves--and no one else can do it for us. Now some may argue that all this sounds like a placebo but that is simply nonsense. The fact is, you can experience medication, or for that matter, any other treatment, and as a result know something happened. Something out of the ordinary. Something not experienced routinely or without the medication or care. This experience effects belief--it's that simple.

Now belief may produce the magic of what many refer to as placebo, or the infamous sugar pill effect. These so-called infamous effects are absolutely real nevertheless. One is not sick and then suddenly well due to the influence of a sugar pill. In the true sense of placebo findings, one is indeed physically ill, their body chemistry proves this; and yet the belief in the "pill" as some new and powerful medication produces a complete reversal in the body. The individual is healed.

To discount such marvelous human abilities with comments like "it only works if you believe it", is to condemn ourselves to a mechanical reality that limits our own ability to experience the full potential of humanness. So remember, good scientific double blind studies, clinical findings and other hard science, that so many of us have to have, show clearly the mind-body reality in wellness and longevity. Adding the power of belief to that science is just what you have been doing with old antiquated versions of the mind-body relationship to health. Each of us can just as well begin today to power the new model, **wellness**, with the same force of belief!

Chapter Twelve

The Pragmatist Within

So from a childhood story of myself to scientific findings with multiple personality patients who display different physiological conditions for each personality, to such miraculous healings as those of the ancient temples of Asclepias with their arts and entertainment programs, to the attitudinal work of men like Jampolski and Cousins, to the viewpoint of such cellular specialists as Lipton, and more, we have looked at the mind-body connection as it relates to wellness and longevity. What can we say for certain? If the fundamental truth of science is that the body is mechanical and works to create health totally **independent** of the mind, then we have a whole lot of interesting phenomena that we are going to have to ignore.

Perhaps some of us will do just that---ignore! Perhaps it's okay to behave as the whimpering shocked dog Seligman discovered in his research. What Martin Seligman of the University of Pennsylvania found was that dogs, conditioned with electric shock under circumstances where they could not escape, did not try to escape when they were shocked in a pen where they could have indeed escaped. They simply accepted the conditioning, and whimpered a lot but made no attempt to help themselves. Dogs that had not been so

47

conditioned would move a few feet, removing themselves from the area where they received the shock. And, as you may have guessed, the animals whose conditioning caused a "helpless" behavior, also experienced a reduction in their immune system. Maybe here we can find a possible explanation for our finding regarding the physician's attitude and the patient's life expectancy. The conditioned patient has become hopeless/helpless just like the shocked whimpering dog. So let's add to our clues, helplessness, or in a positive sense, lack of helplessness.

What would happen if, as the alternative to helplessness, one took the position I did, that of the pragmatist who says, "The proof is in the pudding, and what have I got to lose?" Can we expect to experience a life of health and wellness? What happens if we try accepting the responsibility for our own well-being and ask ourselves simple questions if we sense or feel a sickness coming on? The best three I have found is **"WHAT AM I GETTING OUT OF THIS?", "WHO DO I WISH TO BLAME OR PUNISH,"** and **"WHAT IS THE CONFLICT?"** Now, there are some people that may think a simple question procedure like this one is silly. However, it's amazing the ease with which the answers come, even with the most difficult of diseases. Just by way of example, let me share with you some of the responses I have received from cancer patients in our most recent and current follow up study to this question: **"DO YOU HAVE A BELIEF ABOUT WHY YOU HAVE CANCER?"**

Respondent #1

"I have a history of feeling unworthy, and disappointed in life. I had a miscarriage, my dog was shot six months before my diagnosis, and my daughter decided to live with her father again."

Respondent #2

"I have had breast cancer five times since 1983. Every time I have been under a tremendous amount of stress. Consequently, I believe stress causes cancer in my case."

Respondent #3

"Husband committed suicide 12/83. I had mastectomy 2/84."

Respondent #4

"My brother-in-law has cancer. He is a marvelous teacher and human being. I used to tell God that I'd take his illness if he would make my brother-in-law well. Now we're a two cancer family!"

Respondent #5

"I do not believe I caused the cancer. I have a genetic predisposition according to the experts. Circumstances of my life and subsequent ambivalence about living allowed it to develop and resulted also in a lay period of denial. I finally took action when I found a reason to continue living."

Respondent #6

"Too sensitive, worried too much, felt like a victim when I was married with two children. I couldn't leave. He finally left me. I thought things would get better when we retired. I hated my husband for almost a year approximately twenty-four years ago--my best dear friend (mother) died in 1986. It was terrible!"

Respondent #7

"Family situation which I could not tolerate and had no ability to change: Mother-in-law moved in with us and adult son moved in with us. Mother-in-law ill, adult son depressed, unable to work, and I felt I had no support from husband. I could "feel" myself "dying" a little bit every day."

I came to a point where I decided that maybe I was at least partially responsible for many of my illnesses, especially those pesky regular bouts with sore throats, colds, influenza, etc. As a pragmatist, I decided the proof **was** in the pudding. Maybe I was creating, at some level of my being, discomfort known as illness and then it occurred to me, hey--wait a minute, am I really ready to give up all those comforts that accompany the sickness? All those advantages such as added attention from loved ones, time off with pay while lying around with a good book or a good movie, some soaking in the tub, and doing nothing? Did I really want to give all that up? And then, from answering this type of question, I could see that sickness was not all bad. There were some benefits to being ill!

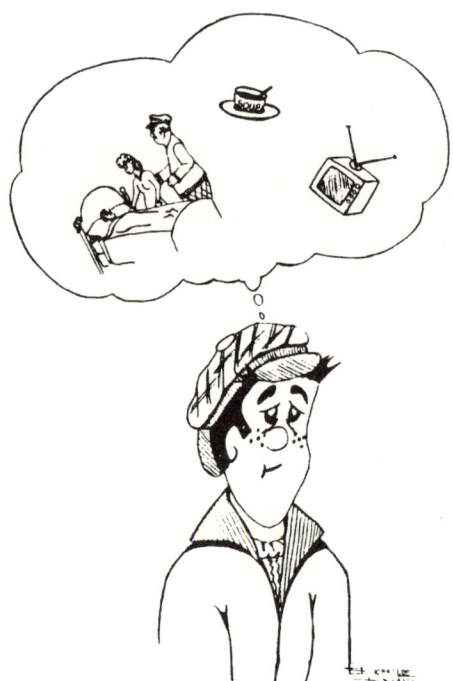

Still, just because one recognizes that there may be benefits from illness, that doesn't mean one can control illness. Or, does it? After all, many of the conflicts dealt with in life get shuffled into matters that become submerged in the subconscious. How can I alter that? How can I take charge of something out of my awareness?

Well, in 1982 I decided to try. I employed what I call the Seven Fundamentals. I share these principles with everyone, in nearly all of my writings and presentations, and later I'll share them with you. Only twice since 1982 have I been ill. In both instances, I was able to source a reason and remember wellness, employ the fundamentals, and leave the illness behind in only a fraction of the time considered normal. In 1982 I decided, just for me, that if I wanted to take a break, to take time off, to bring an end to conflict, to hide from something or someone, to punish myself or others, to get some special attention, and so on, that there were many more productive and fun ways to enjoy these pleasures then getting sick. My annual average of four to six bouts with this and that affliction stopped. That's a lot of remedies that I haven't bought in the past decade. That's a lot of kleenex that I haven't taken to the trash. But this could be a fluke---right? Well, here's another true story that still does not cease to amaze me:

In 1987 a concerned father flew in to see me with a story about his boy, Vic, who was confined to a wheelchair. His father had access to the best of medical care and yet nothing was helping Vic.

Vic had been born with a minor birth defect which was corrected, via a tracheotomy, at the age of two. Soon after he had regained his health a younger sister was born. She, of course, now became the center of attention.

Because illness had provided the means for getting attention from birth until two years of age, and because his present disease started within just a few months after the birth of his younger sister, I theorized that this boy's illness could be his way to regain the attention he had experienced at birth and lost when his sister was born.

With this theory (you can find the case study and details in my book **Subliminal Learning**), we decided to try a subliminal intervention program. We had Vic listen to the subliminal tapes which bombarded his subconscious mind with the idea that he was whole and well. After Vic listened to these tapes for approximately two weeks, and after his subconscious mind had accepted the fact that he was indeed whole and well--guess what? Vic became whole and well. Through the use of these subliminals a true regression in the young man was created, where he returned physically and mentally to the time in his life when he suffered from his birth defect. The regression was so complete that circumstances were created where a second tracheotomy was required. Just as with the first tracheotomy at age two, the surgery was followed by continuing recovery.

Today Vic leads a healthy life. He sent me a photograph that I will always treasure of himself standing beside his new automobile.

Coincidence? A subconscious motive was treated with a subconscious modality -- that of subliminal communication. Even though I witnessed the event, even planned the approach, it still intrigued and amazed me. Is this healing process possible for everyone, I asked? I believe it is.

Chapter Thirteen

The Scientist Emerges

As a scientist, I work to bring information together into a usable formula. I'll try to do that now in simple, straightforward terms. Let's use what we have learned to generate a formula and then make predictions and test our hypothesis.

First of all, what have we learned?

1. Without a doubt, the mind is connected to health. Further, the personality, mood states, and attitude of an individual are related directly to various forms of illness.

2. The amount of responsibility a patient takes for the illness directly relates to recovery.

3. The expectation factor, whether of the physician to the patient or of the patient independent of the health care provider, is directly related to wellness and recovery.

4. For health to be restored, the individual must often return "mentally" to the point before the illness was learned, as in the example of Dr. Milton Erickson or the young man who regressed to the conditions present after his first tracheotomy. **Memories** of wellness are thereby regenerated.

Memory appears to be an all-important factor in wellness. One should be encouraged to remember wellness during any period of disease. In fact, my work has led me to believe that there is a psychological reason behind most diseases. A psychological situation that causes the illness to occur for some reason, even if that reason is self-punishment. And for what it is worth, hypnotic work that has been shown to work for certain diseases, will most certainly work better if it includes regression to the memories of good health as part of the therapy.

In my opinion, then, we could create a formula for the mind's relationship with the body. The formula would use W to represent wellness, E to represent expectation (which is an ever-changing form of true belief) and M to represent memory. Expressed as a formula, $W=EM$, or Wellness equals Expectation multiplied by, or at one with, Memory of wellness. To multiply in this equation, the memory of wellness should be fully brought to mind and placed solidly into expectation.

It may be that the hit-and-miss record of the visualization, or mental imaging process, is due to the ability to remember. Perhaps an artificial experience created during visualization actually becomes real for some because of the inclusion of memory and fails for others because of the absence of enough detail (memory) for it to become real.

These are some of my opinions, but bear with me for a moment.

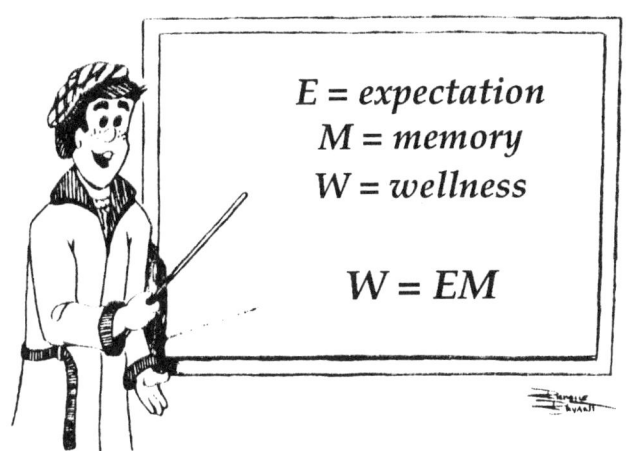

$E = expectation$
$M = memory$
$W = wellness$

$W = EM$

For years I used forensic hypnosis in investigations. On many occasions I saw experiences remembered so completely that it caused a reaction in the body. One such experience I can still see vividly was that of a young man who had been held up at gunpoint. The only thing he could tell the detectives at Sandy City police department following the robbery was that a "very big gun" was shoved in his face. Under hypnosis, I had him replay the incident in his mind, in slow motion, freezing some frames, just as you would on a videotape. In this state of consciousness we were able to obtain detailed descriptions of the suspects and their automobile. But here is my point: when the replay in his mind came to the sequence in which the gun was in the victim's face, I thought his jugular would jump out of his throat. I had to fast-forward the sequence in his mind and assure him that it was only a replay, for it appeared that he could literally have had a heart attack under the stress of the **memory**, for that is indeed what we were dealing with. So when I say revivify a memory, I mean bring it **fully** alive and into the present, just as if it were taking place right now--only make it one of your positive memories!

Alright, so much for what we have learned. This formula has an implicit hypothesis, and that is: within each of us there resides an incredible healing power. To test the hypothesis we can begin as I did, by simply applying the formula in our lives.

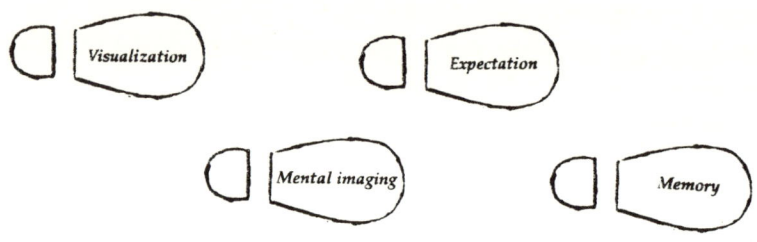

Chapter Fourteen

Owning Your Own Controls

How does one apply our simple formula? Alas, perhaps this question super-imposed on the faces of individuals I have seen suffer with disease, was why the investigator in me was still not satisfied? Why did I feel that a piece of the puzzle was still missing? There were questions still to be answered. For instance, what makes the difference between two children raised in the same environment with the same parents when one ends up a neurosurgeon and the other a hardened violent criminal? What makes the difference between two patients suffering in a hospice center from identical conditions when one requires very little medication and is liked by all, whereas the other suffers bitterly regardless of the medication and is very unpleasant to be around? What are the subtle differences that seem to allow one person to live a certain life-style free of illness, whereas another doing the same things becomes ill as a result? What defines a stimulus as stressful to one while the same exact stimulus is welcomed with excitement by another? To me, the answer was so simple it was overly obvious.

In my work, I have had the opportunity to work with a wide range of individuals in differing settings, ranging from the

57

inmate incarcerated in maximum security to the terminally ill patient in the hospice center. Over the years my observations ultimately led to this hypothesis: the persons who seem to suffer most consider themselves to be victims. The classic victim scenario in the prison generally goes something like this: but for the grace of God, there go you. Translated by the inmate population, this means something like, "What would you do? Where would you be? After all, my daddy was an alcoholic, my mother was a prostitute, and the neighbor boy hung heroin on me when I was only eight."

The fact is, our environment and circumstance do imprint us in profound ways. Our very ability to cope depends in large part on our choices, and they are predetermined in large, by our enculturation process. Thus, what else could the victim of these tragedies do?

We all grow up with some substantially similar ideas and notions about what is fair and acceptable. We all tend to say such things as, "When I'm a parent, I'll do it differently"; and yet, when our children act in some way that meets with our disapproval, we respond just as our parents did. Psychologists call this process imprinting. In very simple terms, if you raise a duckling with chickens, it will behave as a chicken.

A marvelous story illustrates this point:

One day an eagle flew over a chicken coop. To his amazement, pecking in the yard below, was a large gathering of chickens and a lone, beautiful female eagle. He swooped down for a closer look, and the chickens together with the eagle fled to the chicken house. For days the eagle watched the chickens from a distance until one day he was certain that he could stop the beautiful eagle before she reached the chicken house. With the prowess of an eagle, he was suddenly between the eagle and the chicken house. She trembled. He spoke. "What are you doing living down here like a chicken." She answered, "I am a chicken." He argued, showing her the similarities between himself and her. He told her of what it was like to be an eagle and soar high above the earth. His stories only frightened her. Finally she said, "Well, if I'm an eagle, then you will not harm me." He responded in the affirmative. She said, "Then step back and show me." As he stepped back, she ran into the chicken house. When the other chickens questioned her, she told them how she had outsmarted the eagle. Of course, all the chickens commended her for tricking the eagle.

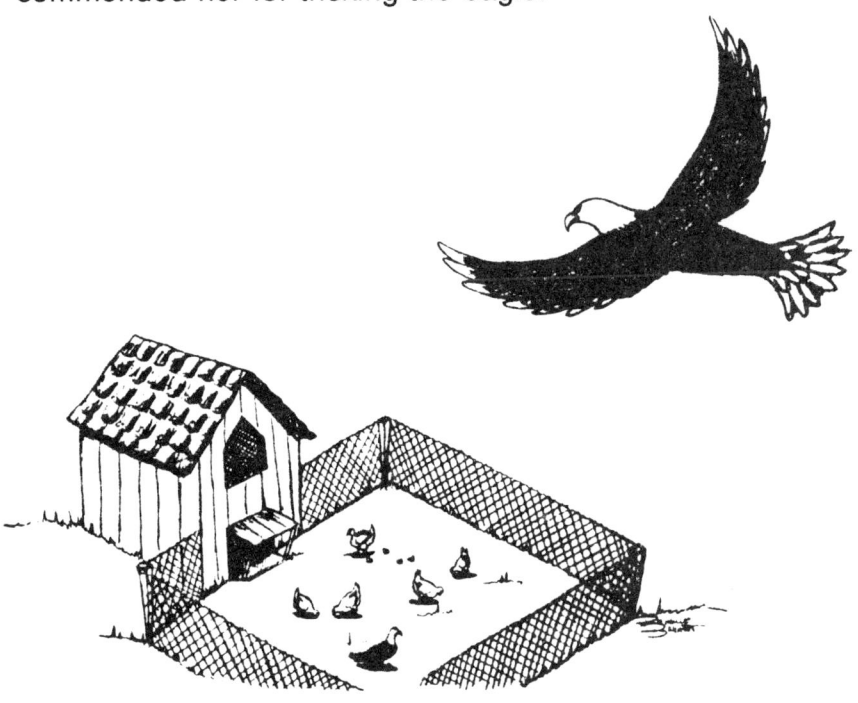

Many of us are like the female eagle. We outsmart ourselves with betrayals of who we really are. Our choices are predicated on our beliefs, and our beliefs have been adopted from the same process inherent to the story about the chickens and the eagle. Here is another example of how this kind of reason pervades who and what we are.

One day a man walking the streets of Manhattan passed beneath a high-rise complex of very expensive condominiums. As he passed under the balcony of one of the two-story units a flower pot that had been placed precariously close to the balcony edge crashed down on his head. Now imagine this man's choices. What could he do? What would be the normal thing to do? He could take the broken pot back to its owners and administer a beating to the idiot that put the flower pot too close to the edge. That's what most people respond with as their first thought when I have presented this scenario to audiences.

What else could he do? He could be metaphysical--you know, kismet, what's to be will be; after all, maybe the blow to his head rearranged some neurons and now he will experience higher consciousness. So be metaphysical, act as if it was supposed to happen, and just go on down the road.

What else could he do? He could be an opportunist. That flower pot fell from a wealthy person's ledge. Whip lash, concussion, something like that---sue the sucker!

What else could he do? How about taking the flower to a florist, repotting it, and returning it as a gift of love? Could he just as well do that?

Of all the possibilities, which one do you think would produce the best outcome for happiness, wholeness, and even health?

The fact is, the normal person has been trained to behave in a normal manner. Normal means that the person has a right to become angry and exact punishment. Robert Laing, in his book **The Politics of Experience,** said that normal man has educated himself to be normal and thus to become absurd. The emotional reaction termed anger is just one such absurdity. What happens to the body when one becomes normal is no less than a weakening of the immune system; further, suspended states of fight or flight, or, as we know it in modern man, anxiety and depression, literally produce chemistry that is toxic to the human condition. As we discussed earlier, these hostile emotions--victim feelings, if you will--literally can condition the body in the direction of disease as well as produce certain diseases in and of themselves.

The correct answer in our flower pot analogy, is of course, repot the flower and return it as a gift. The idea is not foreign as a possible alternative and yet it is seldom ever considered. Our choices arise from our definitions, and they have been incubated all too often in chicken houses. But let's stop for a moment and look at one of the preferred enculturated choices from the human chicken house. My work and research has demonstrated that for every fear there is an anger response. Sometimes the anger is withheld, sometimes it is turned in, and sometimes it is acted out. Nevertheless, there is no such thing as anger without some fear underpinning it! Now, what exactly is anger? My examination of this cycle of fear and anger has given rise to an acronym that I often use when describing anger. A---a, N---nasty, G---getting, E---even,

R---response. A nasty getting even response. If fear and anger are circular, what gives rise to feeling frightened, anxious, or nervous, becoming angry, and then responding in a fight/flight way when the stimulus is something like the way my employer speaks to me, the way my significant other looks at me, or just the stuff one feels when cut off in five o'clock traffic. Not one of these things is truly life-threatening and, after all, isn't that what the fight/flight functions are wired in for, the preservation of the species?

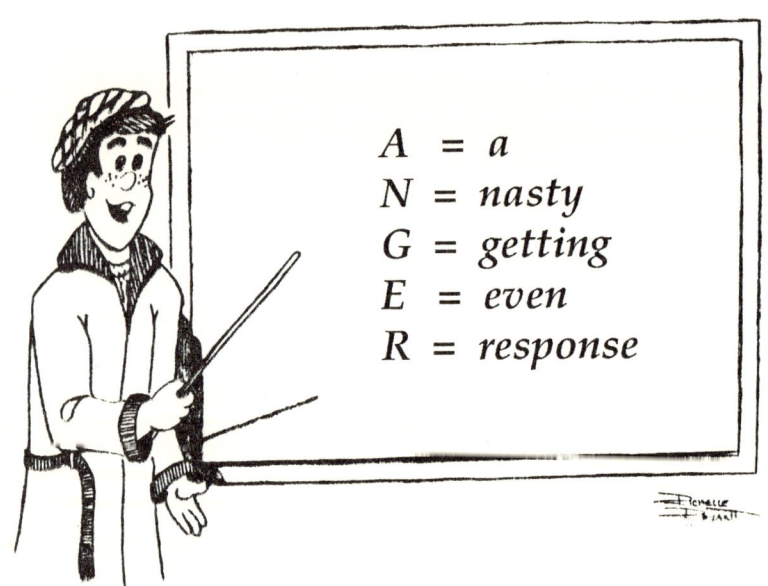

$$A = a$$
$$N = nasty$$
$$G = getting$$
$$E = even$$
$$R = response$$

Dr. Carl LePrecht used to speak of the four drives--the four "F's"-- in his introductory lectures to basic psychology. These four primitive drives were the basis for most behavior. In fact, it was Carl who first suggested to me that perhaps the highest act of human consciousness was cortical inhibition--overriding the wired-in responses that can occur in the primitive brain. The four "F's" are easy to remember because they are oriented to species preservation: fight, flight, feeding, and---well, the propagation of the species.

Why then a fight/flight response to synthetic stimuli--that is, stimuli that are not life threatening? What special lens do we attach to certain events in life that give rise to a perception of threat when indeed the threat is not a tiger in hot pursuit? My early hypothesis regarding the fear/anger loop eventually led me to the conclusion that perceived threats were rejection oriented. In other words, our individual intrinsic value was denied. Interestingly, though, for most of us, the normal strategy for avoiding rejection is itself the ultimate rejection. There are two ways to be tied up in the world. One is to be literally bound with heavy ropes or chains, and another is simply to be tethered to a thread, refusing either to pull hard enough to break it or to let it go. Many of our beliefs are like the thread. We refuse to let them go. Like the eagle raised by the chickens, we know what we are expected to do and define our behavior accordingly. Thus, to resolve conflict we establish strategies designed to protect us from rejection. Among these strategies our defense mechanisms function, as well as our attitudes, toward everything we will ever know in our lives.

When I was a boy my definitions included labels and what I have termed for years as the no-don't syndrome. In my many lectures throughout America and Europe, the audience has repeatedly verified that my experience was not unique. Indeed, it was the rule. If this generalization applies, then most of us were raised with statements like, "You're not old enough," "You're stupid," or "That's stupid," "Children are to be seen and not heard," "Don't do this," "You can't do that," and so forth, as well as a host of labels such as four-eyes, nigger, spick, jew, and so on.

At a very early age I was wearing glasses and my best friend was black. My early definitions were in direct conflict with my experience; still, various strategies for coping with this conflict developed, albeit most unconsciously.

It wasn't until I was in my thirties that I learned that not only did I wear glasses and have black friends, but my grandfather was Jewish and my great-grandmother was Native American. For years I had coped by demonstrating that I was "tough enough" to wear glasses and not get called four-eyes and to stand up for what just inherently seemed wrong and later became known to me as bigotry and racism. In other words, my defense strategy was compensatory--aggression would align my innerself with the outerself. My experience with my training as a child was to avoid conflict by simply becoming too tough for someone to challenge my behavior or too ill to fight.

The result was devastating. Not only did I poison myself but the never ending quest to justify my actions produced increasing needs for aggression. My relationships deteriorated or were destroyed, and--well, you can just imagine the havoc wreaked in my own life. The method of choice for conflict in my particular upbringing was aggressive--and hostility was the norm.

What I have found over the years of life and work is that this was not a unique pattern. Oh, the circumstances may vary from individual to individual, but not the essence of the lesson. The result for many of us is a mechanism called blame. We become helpless victims. It's not our fault. Ah, but remember Seligman's whimpering dogs? Is blame analogous to whimpering? That brings us right back to the prison inmate whose daddy was an alcoholic and so forth. A light went on that set years of work and research into perspective, at least for me.

Now here is the bottom line: as long as individuals blame anything or anyone, they are effectively tied up. There is nothing they can do. They are victims of their circumstances. They can only but whimper. As victims, they are helpless. As victims, perhaps they are even due such benefits as sympathy, attention, special care, and so on. But as victims, they are not in charge of their circumstances or their responses.

Applying this theory, I discovered that regardless of the circumstances, from hospice to prison, the suffering was directly related to blame or "victimhood." What is more, I discovered that on the opposite side of this continuum rested the self-responsible, the person who assumed control of his or her own life and found creative solutions for difficult situations--returning the flower, if you will, replanted in a new flower pot.

These responsible individuals were in charge of their own inner environments. Their secret was simple: they did not become angry and involved in blame. Oh, they did not necessarily accept everyone or anything--in fact, quite the contrary in some instances--but they did not waste time eliminating their possibilities by divesting their power via blame. They took the initiative to resolve situations positively and assumed the responsibility for doing so. Unlike the whimpering victim, they accepted the truth that they were what they made of the stuff of life. (See Appendix A for a self-quiz that may offer you some insight as to your own willingness to accept responsibility).

Again, remember the whimpering shocked dog experiment we discussed earlier? From the results of his experiment, Seligman suggests that many of us have learned that nothing can be done in many circumstances to make a difference. We have already seen that this sense or conditioned belief in victimhood has been demonstrated to affect the immune system in a negative manner. "Nothing I could do"--"helplessness"--"victimhood"--this side of the responsibility equation is among the worst mental processes one can adopt, regardless of its source. Don't forget the results I obtained from the survey of physicians whose patients had used the "Cancer Remission" program. The results of this survey suggested that individuals must fully accept the responsibility for their own lives and mental processes even if that means guarding against the influence of another. I cannot overemphasize this point.

What, then, is the pragmatic way to overcome or, I prefer, to outgrow this early conditioning. Once again, it's so simple as to be difficult--difficult to believe and difficult to do. The answer is, Forgive! In my research we began applying three messages in our tape programs as cognitive tools to untie the victim. They are called the Forgiveness Set and consist of these three statements:

I forgive myself,
I forgive all others, and
I am forgiven.

When you forgive, you cannot blame. If there is no one or nothing to blame, you can't be a victim. If you do not blame, it's exceedingly difficult to become angry. What you cannot become angry about, you do not fear. When there is nothing to fear, there is nothing to become angry about and no one to blame. Life is simply a miracle, and living is the process of maximizing the miraculous experience. Every thought or deed becomes, therefore, differently oriented. When you accept responsibility for everything in your universe, you gain the power to make changes. The real changes are made in you and thus your experience of life and self become qualitatively different almost immediately.

You are in charge of your inner environment, and your beliefs, attitudes, and emotions do matter to you. Your health, your enjoyment of life, your ability to become all that you are is inescapably involved in your ability to forgive and let go.

But, you may say, that's all too simple, and further, life sucks and then we die. I am sure you can find many who will agree. Still, if you want to see the barnyard from the sky, spread your wings, and see for yourself. Seeing is believing. Try it---I promise, you'll like it. And if necessary, fake it until you make it.

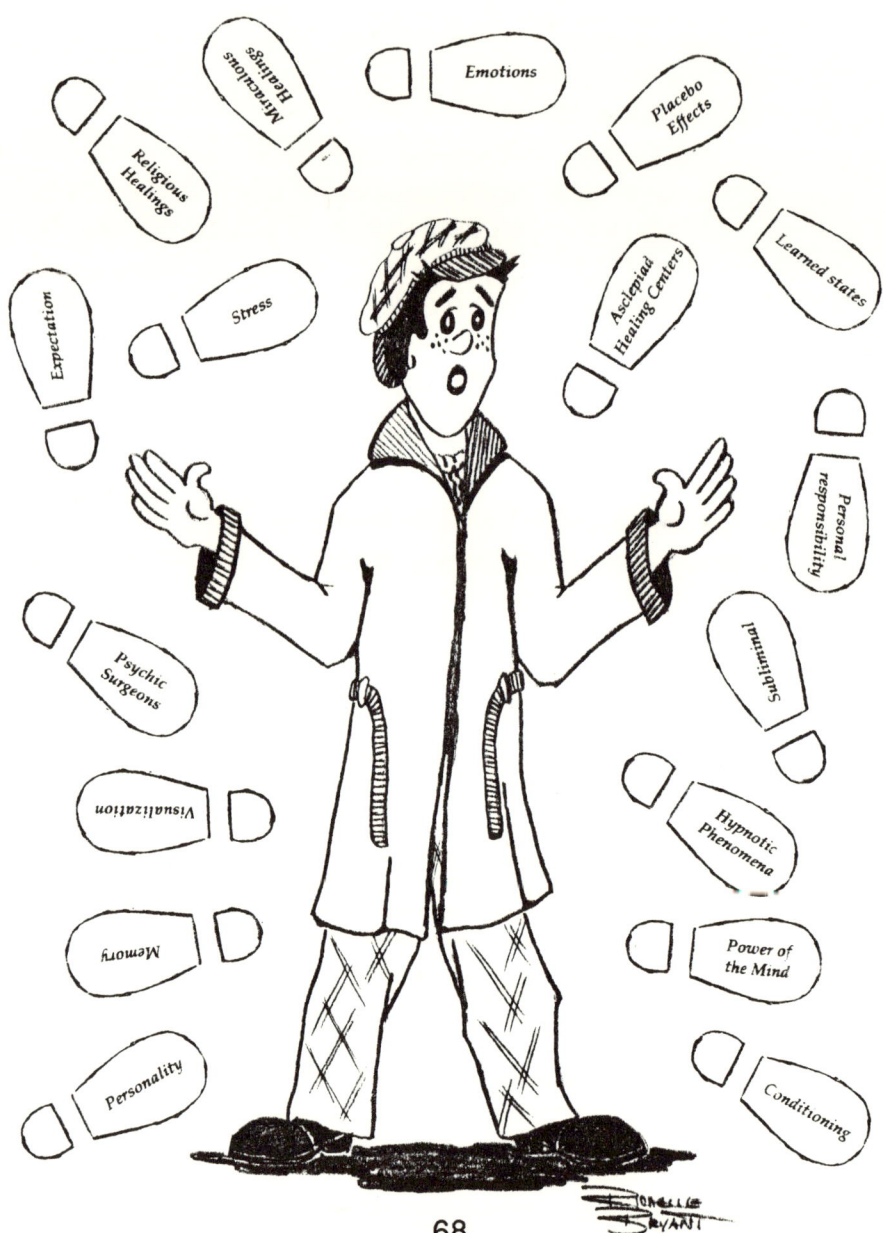

Chapter Fifteen

Making It All Work

With the clues assembled in a simple formula, and now understanding the role of self-responsibility, as far as I am concerned, the case for the mind-body connection is made. But how can we use all of the information obtained to improve the quality of our lives and our health today?

First, pick a time in your life when life was wonderful. You felt great. It was an optimal period of well-being. Remember, this is your memory of a time that you are going to remember and enrich with feelings and emotion appropriate to that time. If you have pictures, recordings, or what-not of that period, get them out and surround yourself with them. I found music selections from the sixties, and the next thing I knew, I was bouncing around like a teenager in the heyday of rock-n-roll. Of course I felt good--every cell in my body was enthused and vital. You try it with your own period of time, but **remember**, choose an optimal period. Merge a few years -- and remember, fully revivify an era where you were at your best!

Second, laugh and smile. Do whatever you need to do. Play old funny movies, watch a standup comic, go to the park and play with your dog, or so on; but laugh. Start by smiling even if you have to force it. The brain doesn't know you are faking the smile. The pure mechanics of contorting the face into a smile causes the brain to release chemicals that naturally improve the way you feel. That is why I said at the conclusion of the last chapter, "So fake it until you make it, if necessary, but smile!"

Third, get some sunlight and fresh air as you did when you were a child. Breathe deeply and evenly. Take a walk, do some exercise, but get outdoors. Remember your youth.

Fourth, and finally, do your emotional work. Let go of blame, shame, guilt, and the like. Be happy. Use the Seven Fundamentals discussed in detail ahead in Chapter 16. Make them part and parcel of your life. They are;
1. You,
2. Thoughts are things,
3. Forgive and let go,
4. Love cancels fear,
5. Acceptance is mastery,
6. Interdependence, and
7. Do it now!

Remember, as long as you blame, you give your power away. Blame provides the excuse that creates victims, who are powerless to do anything because ultimately it is somebody or something else that is at fault. Letting go of these negative feelings empowers you to do, to act, to change. Forgiving and letting go can be as easy as writing a letter, expressing your feelings, ending the letter with something sincere and positive like, "I see good in you," and then disposing of the letter. In other words, if you are angry, you can release the anger and blame in this simple manner without ever confronting the person you're angry with. Forgiving releases you to take control of your life now.

There is also another fun technique you can use. A psychologist friend of mine in Italy, Dr. Monty Renov, suggested to me that I include rhyme in the affirmations used in some of my self-help programs. The theory behind this is simple. Most of us have experienced hearing a song in the morning and having it go round and round in our heads all day. That seems to me to be a pretty effective way of altering self-talk. By altering self-talk, we alter the way we think, which in turn alters the way we view the world, and therefore changes behavior. Since rhyme is what we seem to recall with relative ease, why not replace those old negative thought patterns with something like this:

The thoughts in my mind
Can be endless like time
Why not have the kind
With a helpful rhyme?

Like roses are red
And violets are blue
Life is sure sweet
And living is good too!

Or, up in the morning
And out of the bed
Today is my day
For moving ahead.

I'll do it with vigor
    I'll do it with zest
        I'll know at day's end
            I gave it my best!

All through today
    My strength will prevail
        Within me the **power**
            To create destiny's tale.

So with Love in my heart
    And Life in my hands
        I set my own course
            To magical lands.

And I'll do it with vigor
    I'll do it with zest
        I'll know at day's end
            I GAVE IT MY BEST.

Chapter Sixteen

The Seven Fundamentals

I promised to share with you what I refer to as the Seven Fundamentals. These fundamentals were realized after investigating such questions as, What is success? Why are some people unhappy despite their incomes, possessions, or status? Why do other people seem to have the Midas touch with everything--their relationships, their children, their health, their work, their homes? Why is it that for some, everything works, and for others, nothing works?

Have you ever observed two people with essentially the same opportunities, but one person is happy and the other one is miserable? Isn't happiness the fundamental pursuit of living? Indeed, is it not happiness that constitutes the true meaning of success?

Success is happiness! Truly successful people are happy. Many of their material successes are due to this fundamental secret of the ages: when you are happy and whole in yourself, all good things follow.

Where do happiness and wholeness come from? How does

a person who experiences frustrations in life become whole? If a person becomes whole, will he or she become successful? Can personal wholeness provide happiness, improve self-esteem, and lead to riches and fame, peace, balance, and harmony? Can relationships with family, friends, and associates be improved because one person assumes the responsibility to be personally whole, takes the initiative to exude joy and happiness, seizes the opportunity to empower his or her own life by using the secret of the ages?

The answers to all these questions lie in the Seven Fundamentals of the Master Secret.

Fundamental 1

The first fundamental is **you**, the absolutely awesome and incredible you. Not the you of self-doubt, not the you that fears rejection or failure, not the you that questions your abilities, but the real you. Those other yous are not you. They are synthetic yous built upon limited and false notions of who you are and what you may become. For most of us those false notions originate as we mature. In our very early attempts to achieve acceptance, we often trade off our real selves. The desire to be loved is so strong that many of us give up love or respect for ourselves to obtain security. That trade-off never works, because what we are insecure about in the first place exists within ourselves. The usual response, however, is to find some wise person, guru, or mentor to solve our problems, to show us the way. Consequently the last place we search for serenity, fulfillment, and happiness is within. We are all too often too involved in our out-there search to look within ourselves.

Happiness is a state of mind. The kingdom is within. The real you is a higher you, a higher power that resides within you or is available to you whenever you ask or seek. The fact is, it is your birthright to manifest the glory of the incredible you. You absolutely have the power and ability to experience all the bounties of life, to experience many literal miracles in your life -- for you yourself are a miracle, and all that you are or can ever be is a gift.

So the first fundamental is you. The power resides within you. No one else can do it for you. Your thoughts are reflections of your expectations. What has been sown in your subconscious mind is what you reap. Doubt produces failure, fear yields anger, and belief in limitation is the greatest of all self-fulfilling prophecies.

For eons the sages have advised the development of mind power. All things seem possible for the person who somehow masters this feat. History bears witness to the techniques and teachings that aim solely at controlling the mind to find the higher self within. From yoga to hypnosis, the objective is always first to contact the power within. Some seekers have been successful in contacting that power, but most have met with only partial success. Why? It isn't because the theory is in error or even because the method is necessarily flawed. It is because only you can do it for you. For most seekers, the years of training, the time-consuming rituals, and the rigorous effort ultimately have sufficiently discouraged them, and their attempts have ended in just another failure.

The exploration of the ultimate frontier, the human mind, has changed all of this. Today you can tap your own unlimited potential, creating productive realizations of your real self--the self that you know is inside of you, the self that can succeed and is entitled to joy and happiness. And you can do that in an almost effortless way with many of today's audio and video tools.

The Asclepiads of ancient Greece altered the subconscious language of those whose lives were shallow or incomplete or missing health and happiness by offering experiences that taught the inherent truth: you are what you think yourself to be. Healing and wholeness were restored in Asclepiad centers through realizations that emerged from the language of the subconscious--usually dreams.

Today the advantage of technology makes near-magical visits to the healing centers of well-being possible in your own home and at your own convenience- private, not intrusive, and self-paced. The subconscious beliefs that have programmed you to failure and misery, the subconscious beliefs that fill your mind with self-doubt and fear, can be accessed and changed. Negative subconscious learning can be unlearned, freeing your subconscious mind to create positive acceptances of the real you and thereby liberate you to experience the highest and best of yourself.

Fundamental 2

The second fundamental is that **thoughts are things**. The thoughts we have reveal the beliefs we have about ourselves.

Listen to how we talk to ourselves. Is the language from the inside reflecting optimism, or is it filled with negative and self-limiting ideas? Is luck merely happenstance, or is it mental preparedness meeting opportunity? One of the most successful men in American asks every potential executive this question: Are you a lucky person? If the answer is no, the self-fulfilling prophecy is most definitely true, at least regarding advancement in this executive's empire. So I ask you again: do you consider yourself to be a lucky or an unlucky person? Do you expect good in your life? Do you expect your children to succeed? Your spouse to bring joy to your relationship? Your boss to recognize your efforts? Your fellow workers to admire and respect you? Your neighbors to love you? The guy in traffic to slow down and let you in? Or do you really expect him to flip you off?

What you expect is what you get. Science refers to this phenomenon as the Pygmalion effect. It is a fact: if you expect the worst, you get it. And some of us must love it, because we keep on getting it. Oh, we may complain about it, we may yell and scream when it happens, but what do most of us do about it? Most of us speak and act as though there is absolutely nothing we can do about it. After all, isn't life full of "normal" events that produce "normal" responses? Isn't it normal to become angry for being cut off in five o'clock traffic? Isn't it normal to become fearful when the boss speaks harshly? Isn't it normal to be frustrated with a child's lack of respect or self-responsibility? Isn't it normal to become stuck or just fed up?

Such reactions may be normal, but are they appropriate or conducive to happiness? Has anger ever produced a peaceful sense of harmony within you? Has it ever solved a problem or led to anything other than more anger, guilt, and feelings of being out of control? Such reactions may be normal, but another word for normal is average, which can be defined as the best of the worst and the worst of the best. Neither end of this definition is the highest best of who you really are.

You are your thoughts. You manifest your thoughts, your subconscious beliefs, in everything you experience. Do you believe you deserve happiness, wholeness, and success? You must truly know at all levels of your being that all good things are yours in order for them ever to be yours. You create your own realities. Events are not pivotal points in your life, you are the pivotal point in your life. When your thoughts are in agreement with your desires, your desires will magically materialize.

Fundamental 3

The third fundamental is to **forgive and let go**. That idea may be a bit startling at first, but think about it for a minute. Do you consider yourself to be a victim? A victim of your circumstances? Or are you willing to assume responsibility for who you are? As I stated earlier, there are two ways to be tied up. One is to be tied, literally, by someone else, and the other is to tie yourself, figuratively, by refusing to let go of beliefs that limit your expression of the whole and complete being you are. In other words, as long as you shift responsibility by blaming someone or something for who and what you are, you remove from yourself the power to be anything other than partial and incomplete.

All behavior is the result of choice. Sometimes our choices are made at an unconscious or a subconscious level. For example, we choose to avoid conflict by repressing our true feelings. Later our true feelings become so strong that we can no longer suppress them, and some small incident triggers an overkill response. That is a reactive model- we have lost control. When we assume responsibility for every aspect of our lives, we get in touch with our deepest fears and feelings. The power we gain over our former, reactive behavior provides us with the ability to respond appropriately to all stimuli. That is a proactive model--we are always in control.

The idea was offered earlier that the highest act of consciousness is inhibition of animal stimulus-response conditioning. When we accept responsibility for our every thought and action, we empower ourselves by performing the highest act of consciousness: inhibiting the natural stimulus-response reaction. But that means we no longer have anyone to blame.

In fact, as long as we blame, we effectively eliminate our ability to grow, to be in control, or to experience peace, balance, and harmony. Power to grow resides in forgiveness. Forgiving and letting go will set us free. Forgiving everyone, including ourselves, provides the opportunity to become more than we have been, which for many is but a mere shadow of our real selves. And the irony is that most of us know that we are much more than we have acted out our lives to be!

Fundamental 4

The most powerful force in the world is love. **Love cancels fear**. Fear is the only obstacle that must be overcome in order for all of our experiences to take on new dimensions of meaning and joy. This love is not romantic love between lovers but the unconditional love that we give our children. We are all children in some relative stage of development, learning how to live in joy and happiness. When we truly understand this truth, it becomes easy to forgive another for acts that are selfish and self-centered--and forgive ourselves, as well. "Above all else, respect thyself," said Pythagoras. To love others, we must first love ourselves. We cannot pour from an empty container.

Contemporary studies of behavioral dysfunctions ranging from learning difficulties to criminal activity indicate one common denominator: low self-esteem. Low self-esteem grows out of fear of rejection--rejection by a loved one, an employer, a stranger, anyone who might laugh at our efforts or who would misunderstand or disapprove. On the other hand, high self-esteem grows out of self-acceptance. Self-acceptance is self-love. Self-esteem comes from self-love. We cannot love anyone unless we love ourselves.

Most addictions are the result of low self-esteem and the manner in which we choose to cope with our fears of rejection. Once we get past the inability to love ourselves, we find the ability to love everyone in an unconditional way. That unconditional love does not mean that we necessarily approve of everything everyone says or does, only that we have sense enough to assume responsibility to change what we can change and let be what we cannot change.

When our attitude is one of love, the world fills our lives with others who live the same way. We really do attract others into our lives, almost as if we were mental and behavioral magnets. Suddenly our attitude of love attracts the right people and the right circumstances into our lives, and then the joy, the happiness, and the success we have always been entitled to flourishes.

Loving thoughts breed loving thoughts. Sinister thoughts

breed sinister thoughts. When we desire to be miserable, the last person we seek company with is the one who is happy. The opposite is equally true. Love is indeed the peace that passeth understanding. Love is the creative force of life--and joy, happiness, success, balance, and harmony are its natural fruits.

Fundamental 5

The fifth fundamental is that **acceptance is mastery**. Loving unconditionally suggests accepting others as they are. Furthermore, loving unconditionally suggests accepting yourself as a whole and complete being on the journey of learning we call life.

Acceptance, love, and forgiveness are as necessarily interrelated as each side of a triangle is to the triangle as a whole. Acceptance is the natural process we knew as children. When light faded into night, each of us accepted that this just was the way it worked, and we learned to live accordingly. As we grew older, we began to manipulate our world by means of electricity. Some things in the world can and even should be manipulated to our benefit--turning the dark into a bright space by flipping a light switch may be one of them. But there are other elements in our environment over which we have absolutely no control, nor should we. Attempting to change other people into what we want them to be by manipulating them is what many of us have spent our lives doing.

The best way in which each of us can influence our environment is by example. When we accept other people for who and what they are, we have taken the first step toward accepting ourselves and contributing to the improvement of any condition or situation. Krishnamurti once stated that "you are the world." When we reflect peace and joy from an inner level of being, the world mirrors it back to us. When we judge, condemn, hate, lust, and so on, the world shows us these qualities. The world is a mirror, for the principal function of the world is to provide us the opportunity to learn.

What we resist, we often become. What we like least in another is almost always a reflection of something in ourselves. When we love and accept ourselves, we love and accept others. Each individual who comes into our lives is a teacher. Each has something to contribute to our learning. We in turn have something to contribute to their learning. When viewed from this perspective, our every transaction with another individual transcends the limitations of manipulation.

The fifth fundamental has been called the Golden Rule. Treat others as though they were you, and treat them according to the best **you** there is. Then the rest just happens. What goes out is what you get back. Just as the story in the Bible of the prodigal son teaches us that God has already accepted and forgiven us, so this fundamental suggests that for many of us the least of our brothers and sisters has been ourselves. Accepting and loving ourselves provides the ability to accept and love others, just as accepting and loving others provides the ability to accept and love ourselves.

Acceptance is grace, for acceptance cannot exist without forgiveness and love. With this perspective as the mandate of our experience, we empower ourselves and the world around us. We see clearly that every experience in our lives has occurred to teach us. We can choose to learn quickly and advance, or we can choose to stick around to receive another of those not-so-favored experiences until we do learn. Acceptance will accelerate our personal growth and deeply enrich the quality of every experience.

Thus we all can choose to examine each experience for the good. Just as easily as we can complain and flail about, we can say to ourselves, "I can't wait to find the good in this experience."

This thinking is not crazy or Pollyanna-like. Purely practical logic teaches us that becoming angry or stressful has not and does not produce happiness or joy. As a matter of fact, anger or stress only produces more anger or stress--to say nothing of the toxins such negatives generate in our bodies to slowly poison us.

Fundamental 6

Martin Luther King once said, "I can never be what I ought to be until you are what you ought to be, and you can never be what you ought to be until I am what I ought to be." He went on to say that this mutually related network of reality is the fabric of the human condition.

The sixth fundamental, then, is **interdependence**, the principle that each of us is an aspect of the whole. Each of us invites respect or disrespect according to what we give others, all others. Down through the ages this concept has been given many labels, including the popular label karma. It is called reciprocity. What we sow is indeed what we reap.

Interdependence means individually assuming responsibility

for any condition that is contrary to the quality of humanness in its highest form and then acting to produce, out of the condition or situation, balance and harmony for all. That is not to say that we take up causes and then shove them down someone else's throat. It is to say that we can work in harmony through example and right action to produce an environment that is loving and nurturing for all.

Many people operate in a codependent manner. Their method of assuming responsibility is to manipulate others by placing blame, finding fault, or assuming a contractual posture that goes like this: "If I do this, will you...?" or, "If you loved me, you would..." or, "Don't you feel sorry that I feel..." or, "You need me to...," and so on. Codependence is manipulating another person to provide you with security, sensation, and power. If someone else cannot live or function without you, then your self-worth has been validated--and vice versa. A codependent is a victim, a victim both of his or her surroundings and of other people. The need to control another person is a classic symptom of codependency. Codependency grows out of insecurity. All insecurities are externally oriented. The codependent sees stimuli through the lens of expectation. Expectation is a contract that goes like this: "I will behave this way, if you behave this way;" or, "If you behave that way, I will behave that way." The fear of unfulfilled expectations gives rise to internal conflict.

Happiness is a state of being. It exists moment to moment in the eternal now. If happiness doesn't exist, conflict takes its place, even if the conflict is only the difference between what we think we should be experiencing and we are experiencing. In other words, when we have what we desire, we experience joy. Furthermore, when what we experience is unconditional, as opposed to contractual, then we experience only joy.

Insecurity fuels fear, and fear is a very creative force. What we fear most is therefore very often what we create as our experience. Instead of accepting what is, we project what might be or lament what might have been. We are responsible only for ourselves individually. We must be whole before any event in our lives will be.

Live in the now, for now is really all there ever is. Avoid manufacturing illusions. Where you are is where you are, and that will change only if you do. You, not others, are responsible for your happiness. You are the world!

Fundamental 7

The seventh fundamental is the culmination of all the fundamentals of success. That culminating principle is this: **Do it now!** This is a world of action, not procrastination. For anything to change, you must do the changing. Nothing happens until you make it happen. Only you can do it for you. So do it now.

Most desires for improvements and alternatives for action are relegated to tomorrow--and tomorrow never comes. If you want success, you must act. Success will not just happen. An excellent definition of insanity is doing the same thing over and over again and somehow expecting a different outcome. To get off the path that has never provided happiness, harmony, prosperity, success, peace, or balance, you must get off the path. You must do something different. Not to do so is insane.

Do it now. Each day do what you can do to produce the desired objective, and do it with enthusiasm. Realize that you are in charge and that the fruits of your efforts today will be the food of your being sooner than you might think.

If the world was a world of theory, then none of us would be here. Nothing in this world stands still or waits. No action is inaction. Not to act when an opportunity presents itself is to choose to pass on the opportunity, regardless of its nature. Not to know is one thing; to know and then to do nothing is another. To know but then to fail to do is really a choice that says, "I am already happy with everything; I'm perfect." More power to you if this is so.

If it isn't, then when opportunity knocks, open the door, and be willing to meet opportunity with preparedness. You will soon discover that you are the luckiest person in the world. If you seize every opportunity with a positive expression of joy and a commitment to improve every day in some way, then luck and joy are all that will ever knock.

Do not put off until tomorrow what can be enjoyed today. Follow the Seven Fundamentals, and wisdom will show you the way. You will know what is in your best interest, and if you act, your best interest will be realized. Trust yourself, believe in the incredible you, power your thoughts with desire, accept, forgive, love, let go, and the secret of success will yield its unlimited cornucopia of joy.

Do it, and do it now!

Epilogue

I have had the good fortune as author of this work to benefit from the comments of several readers. Many of them suggested putting note pages at the end of the book since often memories had been provoked during their reading. For example, one reported a competitive rivalry in school with a younger brother. When the younger brother was criticized for under-achievement and poor school work as compared with his older brother, he explained away the problem by blaming it on poor eyesight. His eyesight immediately worsened to near blindness. This condition reversed itself when the two brothers were no longer in the same situation, and today he doesn't even wear glasses. The reader that reported this episode had not seen the connection until he read the book. Often it is easier to see connections of this nature in others as opposed to ourselves. As such, let me suggest that you use the blank pages to jot down examples that you may see in others and then evaluate your own history for such possible connections.

To conclude on a final and humorous note, let me share a letter from actress Linda Hoy, a delightful friend and one of my readers. Linda, like many of us, may have suspected, or even known at some level of her being, how to conduct her life and yet forgets from time to time.

*"First of all, let me say I consider **Wellness: Just A State Of Mind?** to be a blessing, a practical, hands-on, "kick-ass" blessing.*

I had read all but the last four chapters last evening intending to finish reading this morning. Last night I attended a horrendous city council meeting regarding the Performing Arts Center where too little was decided in too long a time. I was tired and awfully fussy this morning - the dog "peed" on my good bed-spread. Oh my, I was blue. I lamented that I was going to be 50 years old this year and couldn't maintain my present job, let alone add to it - starting a theater here in Big Bear. I kicked the dog, slapped the cat and kissed Bill good-bye, then crawled back under "pee" drenched bed clothes with the last four chapters of the book.

And thank goodness I did. It was the wonderful healing I needed. It picked me up by the scruff of the neck, dusted me off, and set me back on the road. It was just what I needed to keep my head afloat long enough for my feet to touch solid ground. And that solid ground was the Seven Fundamentals. I knew this, but I got lost in the drama of "poor me," and lost sight of my goals. My goal to be happy; to be loving; to surround myself with peace and laughter; my goal to lie on my back and watch the clouds go by, to run and fall down in the leaves.

Thank you.

I want to own this book. I want to have one in my purse, one on my bed-stand and several to send to friends.

Thank you again,

Linda Hoy

Notes

Notes

Notes

Notes

Notes

Notes

Notes

Notes

Notes

Recommended Readings

Brain Mind Bulletin, 2, 4d. Bodymind Update: Cancer, Alcohol & Pot, Psychosis.

Brain Mind Bulletin, 2, 15b. Grief Lowers Immune Response in Study: Stress Precedes Onset of Disease.

Chopra, D. (1989). Quantum Healing: Exploring The Frontiers of Mind/Body Medicine. Bantam Books.

Cohen, S. (1991). Emotional Stress Linked to Common Cold. **Science News, 140**, no. 9.

Jampolski, G. (1981). Love Is Letting Go of Fear. Bantam Books.

Jampolski, G. (1983). Teach Only Love. Bantam Books.

Krasner, A.M. (1990). The Wizard Within. ABH Press.

Krieger, D. (1975). Hospital Study: "Therapeutic Touch" Affects Hemoglobin. **Brain Mind Bulletin, 1,** no.2c.

Laurence, J.R. & Perry, C. (1988). Hypnosis, Will & Memory. Guilford Press, U.K.

Lipton, B. (1991). Private communication.

Locke, S., Colligan, D. (1986). The New Medicine of Mind and Body. E.P Dutton.

Maltz, M. (1969). Psycho-Cybernetics. Pocket Books.

Ornstein & Sobel (1987). The Healing Brain. Simon & Schuster.

Posner, J. (1990). Private communication.

Putnam, F. (1987) Noetic Sciences.

Rossi, E.L. (1986). The Psychobiology Of Mind-Body Healing. W.W. Norton.

Siegel, B. (1988). Love, Medicine & Miracles. Caedmon.

Simonton, C. (1976). Simonton's Report on 110 Cases: Imagery Therapy Can Retard Cancer. **Brain Mind Bulletin, 1,** no. 23c.

Simonton, C. (1991). Getting Well Again. Rev. ed. J.P. Tarcher, Inc.

Taylor, E. (1988). Subliminal Learning: An Eclectic Approach. R K Book. Big Bear City, CA.

Udolf, R. (1981). Handbook of Hypnosis for Professionals. Van Norstrand Reinhold Company.

Appendix A

SELF-RESPONSIBILITY QUIZ

Read the questions below and answer them as truthfully as possible according to Never, Sometimes or Usually. Think your responses through carefully before answering.

	NEVER	SOMETIMES	USUALLY
1) Do you believe that you are a lucky person?			
2) Do you worry about what others think of you?			
3) Do you fantasize about hurting someone?			
4) Do you like violent movies?			
5) Is it easy to accept others mistakes?			
6) Do you dwell on negative experiences?			
7) Do you look forward to a very long life?			
8) Do you make enemies?			
9) Do you blame anyone for your circumstances?			
10) Do you like your work?			
11) Do you look forward to life?			
12) Do you fear death?			
13) Do you take good care of yourself?			
14) Do you like your body?			
15) Do you consider yourself fortunate?			
16) Do you blame yourself?			
17) Do you blame others?			
18) Do you pity people?			
19) Do you feel sorry for others?			
20) Does the weather upset you?			
21) Do you get angry?			
22) Do you yell at others?			
23) Does risk frighten you?			

	NEVER	SOMETIMES	USUALLY
24) Do delays frustrate you?_____			
25) Does health worry you?_____			
26) Does living excite you?_____			
27) Do you wish you could get even with someone?_____			
28) Has someone stopped you from good things?_____			
29) Do you deserve more?_____			
30) Do you begrudge others?_____			
31) Are you jealous?_____			
32) Are you deserving?_____			
33) Does your work anger you?_____			
34) Do others aggravate you?_____			
35) Do you like yourself?_____			
36) Does pain usually frighten you?_____			
37) Does illness scare you?_____			
38) Are you happy?_____			
39) Do you get along with others?_____			
40) Does losing upset you?_____			
41) Do you wish you were different?_____			
42) Is life too good to you?_____			
43) Do you make friends easily?_____			
44) Is it important to be right?_____			
45) Do you lie to others?_____			
46) Do you exaggerate your experiences?_____			
47) Do you love easily?_____			
48) Do you like learning?_____			
49) Do you enjoy new experiences_____			
50) Do you look forward to new adventures?_____			

SCORING INSTRUCTIONS

A. Add up the total "S" answers x 1 point and subtract from 100.

B. Count "U's" for questions:
    3, 4, 6, 8, 9, 12, 16 through 25, 27, 28, 30, 31, 33, 34, 36, 37 40,41, 42, 44, 45, 46 x 2 point and subtract from remainder of A.

C. Count "N's" for questions:
    1, 2, 5, 7, 10, 11, 13, 14, 15, 26, 29, 32, 35, 38, 39, 43, 47, 48, 49 & 50 x 2 point and subtract from remainder of B.

RESPONSIBILITY SCALE EVALUATION TABLE

RAW SCORE	INTERPRETATION
80 or higher	This subject is in charge of their life and usually will not experience seasonal illness or other psychologically aggravated diseases. A score of 80 or more should also be evaluated for denial. Life circumstances, health and pain thresholds will reveal whether a score of 80 or more is indicative of self responsibility/control or other mechanisms including dishonest answers.
70 to 80	This subject normally is in control, capable of high pain thresholds, finds life invigorating, is optimistic and generally loves living.
60 to 70	Normally this subject is tending toward "self actualizing" goals. They are probably working on personal growth and/or growing through trauma or catastrophe. Their outlook on life tends toward self guidance but they are not ready to accept the idea that they indeed are the fabric of their responses to life's stimuli.
50-60	This subject wishes to believe that they can change their circumstances but is

not willing to give up the traditional victim role.

49 and lower For this subject, the world acts on them and they can only respond. They will have mechanistic views of life, health and so forth. They are victims in a hostile environment.

Special note: This is an experimental evaluation instrument. This instrument is provided to you with the hope that you will share your experiences and data arising from its use. The utility of this instrument is entirely contingent upon the treatment theory advanced by the author. Said treatment theory proposes that suffering is directly related to the victim/responsible scale and to the precise extent that one assumes responsibility for their lives the quality of their experience is enhanced, thereby influencing health, pain thresholds, social adjustment in general, relationships, self-esteem and so forth. We hope you find the instrument together with the treatment protocol useful and empowering.

OTHER BOOKS BY ELDON TAYLOR

Subliminal Learning $12.95
Subliminal Communication $8.95
Subconscious Surgery $17.95

Simple Things and Simple Thoughts $8.95
The Little Black Book $1.50
Exclusively Fabricated Illusions
     (loose leaf work book $14.95

For more information regarding these books and the many self-help audio programs by Eldon Taylor, send for our **FREE** catalog:

R K Book
816 W. Big Bear Blvd.
Big Bear City, CA
92314